# Fundamentals for Cosmetic Practice
## Toxins, Fillers, Skin, and Patients

Michael Parker, BSc MBBS FRCR

*With illustrations by Charlie James*

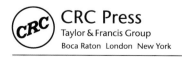

**CRC Press**
Taylor & Francis Group
Boca Raton  London  New York

CRC Press is an imprint of the
Taylor & Francis Group, an **informa** business

First edition published 2022
by CRC Press
6000 Broken Sound Parkway NW, Suite 300, Boca Raton, FL 33487–2742

and by CRC Press
2 Park Square, Milton Park, Abingdon, Oxon, OX14 4RN

© 2022 Taylor & Francis Group, LLC

*CRC Press is an imprint of Taylor & Francis Group, LLC*

*Library of Congress Cataloging-in-Publication Data*
Names: Parker, Michael (Michael James), author.
Title: Fundamentals for cosmetic practice : toxins, fillers, skin, and patients / by Michael Parker.
Description: First edition. | Boca Raton : CRC Press, 2022. | Includes bibliographical references and index. |
    Summary: "Many medical professionals are now seeking to train in Cosmetic Practice, and there are many
    courses offering practical training and many texts offering detailed guides to the procedures; this text offers
    instead a helpful overview of the fundamentals involved and how they impact on practical skills, patient
    management, and potential complications. It constitutes the perfect guide to professional certification and beyond
    that to Cosmetic Practice. Presents the starter in aesthetic practice with the fundamentals of minimally invasive
    treatments. Offers a reliable resource for any medical professional wishing to certify in this specialty. Combines
    material on both main treatment and on aesthetic patient management"—Provided by publisher.
Identifiers: LCCN 2021044898 (print) | LCCN 2021044899 (ebook) | ISBN 9781032057163 (hardback) |
    ISBN 9781032057125 (paperback) | ISBN 9781003198840 (ebook)
Subjects: MESH: Mesotherapy—methods | Mesotherapy—adverse effects | Dermal Fillers—therapeutic use |
    Botulinum Toxins—therapeutic use | Physician-Patient Relations
Classification: LCC RL120.B66 (print) | LCC RL120.B66 (ebook) | NLM WO 595 | DDC 615.7/78—dc23
LC record available at https://lccn.loc.gov/2021044898
LC ebook record available at https://lccn.loc.gov/2021044899

ISBN: 978-1-032-05716-3 (hbk)
ISBN: 978-1-032-05712-5 (pbk)
ISBN: 978-1-003-19884-0 (ebk)

DOI: 10.1201/9781003198840

Typeset in Times
by Apex CoVantage, LLC

Printed in the UK by Severn, Gloucester on responsibly sourced paper

 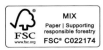

*Dedicated to my darling Rhianna, without whom I would have never even embarked on this journey*

# Contents

# Acknowledgements and Preface

## ACKNOWLEDGEMENTS

With special thanks to Dr Rhianna Davies, Dr Robert Mooney, and Dr Nathalie Boulding for their contributions to this text.

## PREFACE

Medical aesthetics is a rapidly expanding industry worth over £3.6 billion in the United Kingdom. There is no shortage of consumers seeking non-surgical cosmetic procedures, and there are more people than ever seeking to be trained to perform them.

I have found my time performing non-surgical cosmetic procedures to be thoroughly enjoyable, as it has been a nice change to give patients what they *want* as opposed to what they *need*, which is not often the case in conventional medicine. Being able to help individuals elevate their self-esteem is an incredible privilege and not something which should ever be taken for granted.

After spending many years practising in botulinum toxin and dermal fillers, I became all too aware that many individuals (including myself when I trained) are not being taught the ins and outs of cosmetic practice in sufficient depth. The rise of the "one-day course" has led to a false sense of security in newly qualified practitioners with at times devastating results. I was one of those people when I first started my practice, and it soon dawned on me that I had nobody to call for help should a complication arise. It was the absolute definition of *sink or swim*. To try to protect my patients (and my medical licence!) I spent my evenings reading and making notes to try to become a safe and effective practitioner. This book is a culmination of my research.

Please note: This book does not constitute formal medical advice and it is the duty of the practitioner reading it to double-check any information within it with other sources as well as using their own clinical judgement. This book is intended to be read by qualified medical professionals alongside formal, practical training in botulinum toxin and dermal fillers. This book should in no way be interpreted as a substitute for formal training in this field. The author accepts no responsibility to harm to persons or property arising from or related to the use of material within this book.

# 1 The history of botulinum toxin

In 1820, a German medical officer, Justinius Kerner, first described the effects of botulism after systematically observing the effects of the disease then known as "sausage poisoning". He discovered through numerous experiments on both himself and animal models that botulinum toxin would interrupt somatic (conscious motor) and autonomic (unconscious) nerves without having any impact on the sensory or cognitive functions of the individual tested.

Seventy-five years later in 1895, Professor Émile van Ermengem identified *Clostridium botulinum* as the causative organism for the disease botulism after 34 funeral attendees were noted to develop symptoms of this disease after eating partially salted ham. Professor van Ermengem discovered that extracts from the ham served at the funeral induced botulism-like symptoms in laboratory animals, allowing the link to be made between this bacterium and disease.

The medical implications of botulinum toxin were first successfully utilised in the 1970s by Dr Alan Scott. His initial studies on primates revealed that injecting mere picograms of the toxin into the muscles around the eye caused long-lasting paralysis with no significant side effects. After securing a licence from the US Food and Drug Administration (FDA), Dr Scott began to produce botulinum type A neurotoxin in a lab in San Francisco. He hypothesised it may work for strabismus, and subsequently proceeded to treat his first patient with this condition with Botulinum toxin in 1977 before publishing his results in the journal of the American Academy of Ophthalmology in 1980. He named the botulinum toxin he had synthesised *Oculinum*, or "eye-aligner".

The cosmetic implications for botulinum toxin were identified in the late 1980s by Dr Richard Clark, who had a patient who had sustained paralysis of one of the nerves of their forehead following complications during a facelift. He was aware that the nerves may take up to two years to fully regenerate and therefore did not want to perform any further surgical interventions until this time had elapsed. Dr Clark was aware of the previous work by Dr Scott and others in using botulinum toxin in the treatment of strabismus and facial tics and supposed that it may also work in smoothing forehead wrinkles. After achieving FDA approval, Dr Clark successfully treated his patient in 1989 and published his results in the *Journal of Plastic and Reconstructive Surgery*. The work of Dr Clark was further developed by a husband-and-wife duo, Dr & Dr Carruthers, one a dermatologist and the other an ophthalmologist, who successfully used botulinum toxin to treat the glabellar complex, the primary muscle group of the face involved in frowning. Their research was first published in 1992.

After further extensive research, the FDA gave a licence for the use of botulinum toxin A to treat the glabellar complex, and its cosmetic use has continued to grow. At

DOI: 10.1201/9781003198840-1

present, it is frequently used in cosmetics to treat forehead wrinkles, frown lines and "crow's feet" around the eyes. See Figure 1.1.

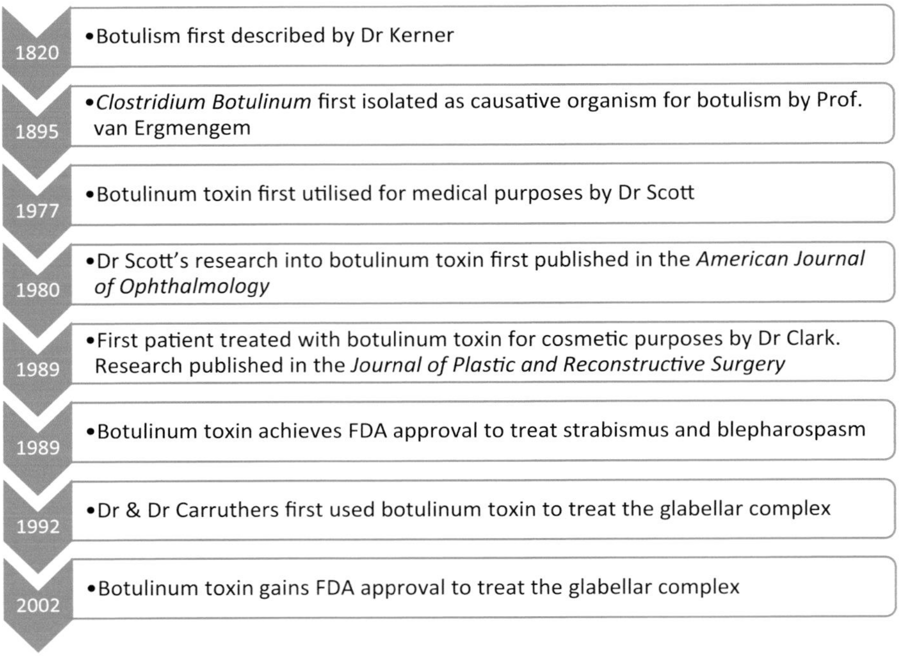

| 1820 | • Botulism first described by Dr Kerner |
| 1895 | • *Clostridium Botulinum* first isolated as causative organism for botulism by Prof. van Ergmengem |
| 1977 | • Botulinum toxin first utilised for medical purposes by Dr Scott |
| 1980 | • Dr Scott's research into botulinum toxin first published in the *American Journal of Ophthalmology* |
| 1989 | • First patient treated with botulinum toxin for cosmetic purposes by Dr Clark. Research published in the *Journal of Plastic and Reconstructive Surgery* |
| 1989 | • Botulinum toxin achieves FDA approval to treat strabismus and blepharospasm |
| 1992 | • Dr & Dr Carruthers first used botulinum toxin to treat the glabellar complex |
| 2002 | • Botulinum toxin gains FDA approval to treat the glabellar complex |

**FIGURE 1.1**    Timeline of botulinum research and practice.

# 2 The history of dermal fillers

The success of botulinum toxin for treating fine lines and wrinkles in the upper face demanded a product of similar efficacy to treat age-related changes of the lower face. Consumer desire for office-based procedures with minimal downtime and side effects has driven innovation in the field of dermal fillers. For a product to be acceptable to both patient and physician, it needs to be safe, effective, convenient, and affordable. The side effects must be minimal, the pain must be tolerable, and the results need to be of a predictable duration, with straightforward storage, preparation and administration. At present, there are in excess of 35 companies producing dermal fillers worldwide, offering a range of choice to both practitioners and consumers. The myriad of dermal fillers available for purchase allows practitioners to select dermal fillers with the appropriate qualities to create their desired cosmetic outcomes.

The use of dermal fillers began in 1893, when a German physician, Dr Franz Neuber transplanted endogenous fat from the arms of patients to their faces to fill defects and reconstruct scars. The first exogenous cosmetic injectable was paraffin in the late 1800s; however, this was soon abandoned due to significant complications including embolisation, migration and granuloma formation. From the 1940s to the 1950s, silicone was used as a dermal filler agent; however, it was never approved by the FDA for facial augmentation. It was inevitably banned as an exogenous dermal filler in 1992 due to its side-effect profile, including silicone embolism syndrome and the formation of nodules and granulomata due to the host's response to foreign bodies. Silicone embolism syndrome was arguably the most serious potential side effect of the use of this filler, presenting with shortness of breath, hypoxia, haemoptysis and proving fatal in up to one-quarter of patients affected.

Next, in the 1970s, came animal-based collagen derived from calfskin. Bovine collagen was used to correct acne and pockmarks, lipoatrophy in HIV and soft-tissue augmentation of the lower face. Zyderm® and Zyplast®, manufactured by Allergan, were produced by Stanford University and approved by the FDA in 1981, becoming the first injectable formally approved for soft-tissue augmentation. These were, on the whole, well tolerated, yet as the tissue is foreign to that of the host, skin testing for sensitivity had to be carried out pre-treatment to decrease the risk of hypersensitivity reactions. The need for skin testing and limited duration of action restricted the popularity of bovine collagen; however, it remained the only approved injectable filler for over 20 years until the development of the first human-derived bioengineered collagen fillers in 2003: Cosmoplast® and Cosmoderm®. These agents had the advantage of not requiring skin testing as they are human-derived products and subsequently confer a very low risk of hypersensitivity reactions. More recently, autologous collagen filler has been used, harvested from the patient during elective surgery, for example Autologen®, developed by the Collagenesis corporation. These

DOI: 10.1201/9781003198840-2

fillers also have a relatively short duration of action of approximately seven months, and when paired with the need for surgical procedures to obtain them, they have not garnered much popularity.

December 2003 signified the arrival of hyaluronic acid (HA) fillers, which have both a longer effective timespan and more tolerable side effect profile in comparison to collagen fillers. The first FDA approved HA filler was Restylane®, produced by Galderma. HA can be animal or non-animal derived and is a naturally occurring polysaccharide found throughout cutaneous tissues, making allergic reactions *theoretically* impossible. HA fillers can be used for cosmetic augmentation, filling of defects, and softening wrinkles. Their plumping effects are in no small part due to their hydrophilic properties, and they also may confer longer-term effects due to neocollagenesis. The next HA filler to be developed, Perlane®, was a more viscous form of Restylane and was approved for use by the FDA in 2007. Restylane® and Perlane® are non-animal derived HA fillers synthesised by cultures of the bacteria *Streptococcus equii*. Another commonly used HA dermal filler is Juvederm®, produced by Allergan and first released in September 2006.

The main limitation of HA fillers is their relatively short duration of action when compared with permanent fillers, which is discussed later. They do, however, have the advantage of being dissolvable by hyaluronidase if the effect is undesirable or should complications occur. The decision to add lidocaine to the product for local anaesthesia revolutionised patient comfort and the tolerability of dermal filler treatments. The first dermal filler to include lidocaine was created by Anika Therapeutics and named Elevess®. It is a non-animal-derived product and, at the time of writing, has the highest concentration of HA available in a commercial filler. More recent products such as Puragen® use double-cross-link technology reducing the rate of degradation and increasing their ability to add volume.

Formulations of non-permanent dermal filler which are not HA based include poly-L-lactic acid (PLLA) and calcium hydroxyapatite (CaHa). PLLA was first licensed by the FDA in 2009 under the trade name Sculptra®. These fillers are broken down over an average of nine months to two years after administration; however, their cosmetic effects often last longer than this due to stimulation of neocollagenesis through activation of dermal fibroblasts. CaHa fillers are made up of microspheres which illicit minimal foreign body reaction, do not migrate within tissues and trigger neocollagenesis alongside their volume-enhancing effects. As it is a more viscous filler, CaHa is primarily designed for use in deeper soft tissues, such as the cheeks. See Figure 2.1.

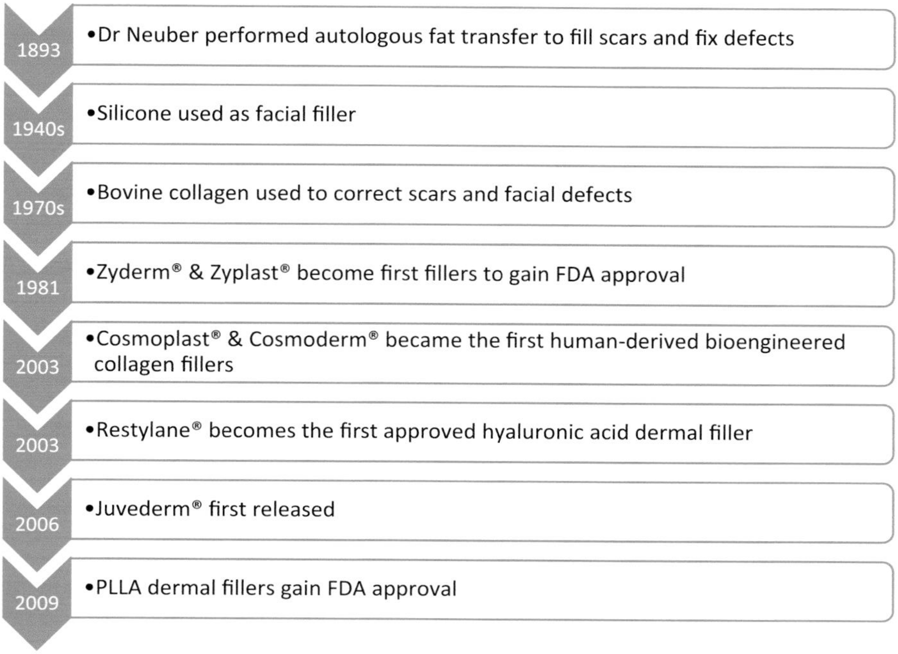

**1893** •Dr Neuber performed autologous fat transfer to fill scars and fix defects

**1940s** •Silicone used as facial filler

**1970s** •Bovine collagen used to correct scars and facial defects

**1981** •Zyderm® & Zyplast® become first fillers to gain FDA approval

**2003** •Cosmoplast® & Cosmoderm® became the first human-derived bioengineered collagen fillers

**2003** •Restylane® becomes the first approved hyaluronic acid dermal filler

**2006** •Juvederm® first released

**2009** •PLLA dermal fillers gain FDA approval

FIGURE 2.1   Timeline of dermal fillers research and practice.

# 3 Facial anatomy

Before treating a patient with botulinum toxin or dermal fillers, it is essential to understand exactly *where* you are inserting your needle and *why* you are aiming for that particular part of the face. As you progress through your training and develop your practice, you will find that more often than not, your anatomical knowledge is crucial for safely administering treatments and for working out *how* to treat your more complex patients. In this section, we cover the relevant musculoskeletal anatomy of the face, the nervous and arterial supply and venous and lymphatic drainage. Gaining an intimate knowledge of these complex anatomical structures will give you a solid foundation to treat your patients safely and effectively in the future.

## FACIAL BONES

Before considering the soft tissues of the face, one must first gain an appreciation of the bones to which they are attached. The bones not only offer protection to the eyes and brain, but also give structural support to the muscles and vasculature of the face itself. The true facial skeleton is made of fourteen bones; however, we shall also include the frontal bone in our discussion of facial osteology for practical purposes – bringing our number of bones up to fifteen.

The bones of the face (Figure 3.1) include the following:

- *Frontal bone*, the bony part of the forehead
- *Sphenoid bone*, the lateral portion of which can be demonstrated inferior to the frontal bone, anterior to the temporal bone and superior to the zygoma
- *Temporal bones*, lateral to the frontal bones and comprise the area colloquially known as the temple
- *Nasal bone*, unsurprisingly the bony portion of the nose
- *Maxilla*, the bone inferior to the orbits, medial to the zygoma and lateral to the nasal bone
- *Zygoma*, the bones which make up the lateral most aspects of the cheeks
- *Mandible*, colloquially known as the jawbone

Now that we have an appreciation of general osteology of the anterior skull and face, it is important to understand the specific function and anatomical locations of each of these bones to allow safe cosmetic practice. In the remainder of this chapter, we discuss the individual bones of the face, their functional anatomy and their relevance to common cosmetic procedures.

DOI: 10.1201/9781003198840-3

## FRONTAL BONE

The frontal bone (Figure 3.2) is technically one of the bones of the skull as opposed to one of the bones of the face. Although any true anatomists will be undoubtedly displeased with it being discussed in the context of facial osteology, when considering

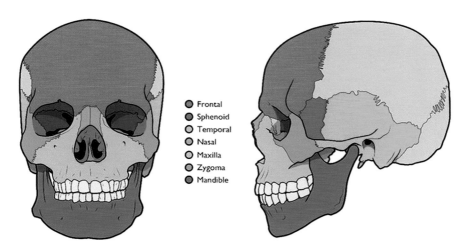

Frontal
Sphenoid
Temporal
Nasal
Maxilla
Zygoma
Mandible

FIGURE 3.1    The bones of the face.

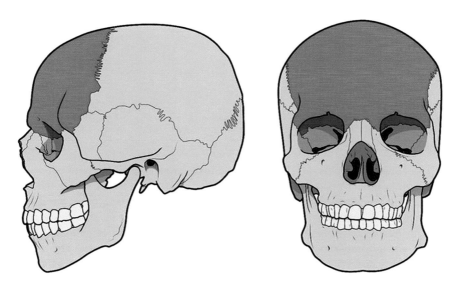

FIGURE 3.2    The frontal bone.

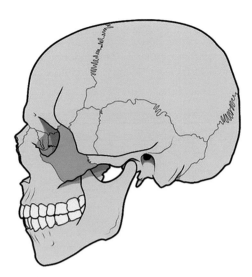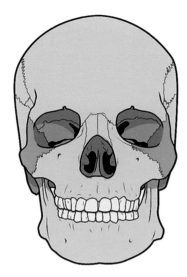

**FIGURE 3.3**  The zygoma.

dermal filler and botulinum toxin administration it is of key importance in both the assessment of the face and administration of treatments.

The frontal bone is the bone of the forehead and is formed of two distinct parts: the *squamous* part, which is the flat piece of bone which makes up the forehead, and an *orbital* part, which comprises the roof and medial aspect of the eye socket. The frontal bone technically has 12 bony articulations; with the four primary *facial* articulations as follows:

- Superiorly: Parietal bone
- Laterally: Zygoma
- Inferiorly: Maxilla
- Medially: Lacrimal bone

### Zygoma

The zygoma is the cheekbone (Figure 3.3) and is therefore a very important bone when it comes to beauty. It sits proud on the upper lateral part of the face, forming the bony prominence of the cheek as well as the lateral wall of the orbit. The zygoma has a *body*, the palpable bony protuberance you can feel when you press on your cheek which articulates with the maxilla, an *arch* which extends posteriolaterally and attaches to the temporal bone; and a *frontal process* articulates superiorly with the frontal bone. The zygoma not only offers protection to the cheek and globe but also offers attachments for many muscles of the face, which are discussed in greater detail in the facial muscles chapter.

### Maxillae

The maxillae are the bones which form the medial aspect of the cheek (Figure 3.4), positioned between the nasal bone and zygoma. They have three primary functions:

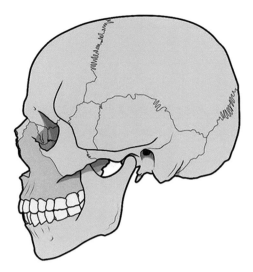
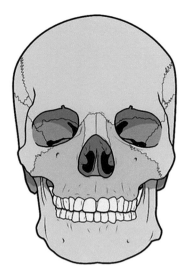

**FIGURE 3.4**  The maxillae.

1. Allowing a point of anchor for the upper teeth in the *alveolar process*
2. Forming the floor and lateral wall of the nasal cavity
3. Forming part of the medial wall of the orbit

The point of fusion of the maxillae is at the midline immediately inferior to the nose at the *intermaxillary suture*. Aside from structural support, the maxillae contain sinuses which are important in both altering the depth of voice as well as keeping decreasing the weight of the facial bones. The maxilla is also the site of the infra-orbital foramen, which is located just below the infraorbital margin of the orbit, at an average distance of 6–10 mm inferiorly in the midline. The infraorbital fora-men is important in the transmission of the infraorbital artery, vein and nerve, and therefore, this region must be respected, especially in the context of dermal filler administration as it is at risk of avascular necrosis, filler embolisation and neuronal damage.

Nasal bones

The nasal bones are paired bones which form the bony portion of the nasal bridge (Figure 3.5), found in the midline in the upper part of the face. The superior portion of the nasal bone is covered by the *procerus* and *nasalis* muscles. The nasal bones articulate with the frontal bone superiorly, the maxillae laterally and the ethmoid bones posteriorly. They are punctured at multiple sites by tiny foramina which allow for veins to exit the skull. Great care must therefore be taken when administering filler for non-surgical rhinoplasty due to the significant risk of venous ischaemia at this point.

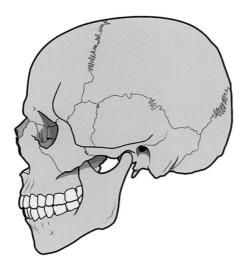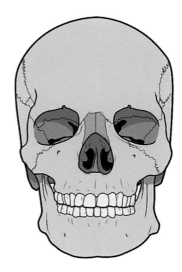

**FIGURE 3.5**   The nasal bones.

MANDIBLE

The mandible is the jawbone (Figure 3.6), and it articulates with the temporal bone at the *temporomandibular joint*, allowing us to open and close the mouth at our leisure. It is found directly inferior to the maxilla and offers a point of anchorage of our lower teeth. The mandible is a complex bone with multiple discernible anatomical segments, including the body, angle, ramus, condyle and coronoid process. The area at which the two halves of the mandible fuse during development is known as the *symphysis menti*, located in the midline of the chin. The mandible has two main foramina on each side, the *mandibular* and *mental* foramina. The mandibular foramina are located in the middle of each mandibular ramus, and the mental foramina are located just lateral to the chin bilaterally. The mental foramina are of key clinical significance regarding augmentation of the chin with dermal fillers, as with any other facial foramina, due to the risk of avascular necrosis, filler embolisation and neuronal damage of structures exiting them.

## FACIAL FORAMINA

The reason why understanding facial bony anatomy is important is not just due to the bones themselves, but also their *foramina*. Foramina are holes in bone which allow for the passage of contents from within a bony cavity (such as blood vessels and nerves) to the outside world. The foramina of the face permit the transmission of nerves, arteries and veins in and out of the safety of the skull to allow them to innervate, supply, and drain the overlying soft tissues (Figure 3.7). A lack of knowledge of the location and function of the key facial foramina can result in serious harm to a patient during the administration of dermal fillers and botulinum toxin.

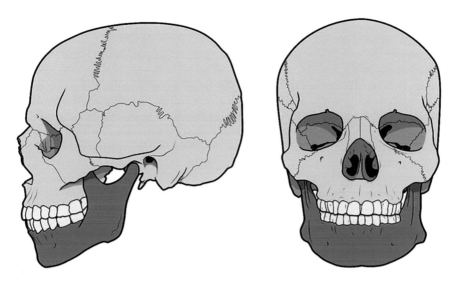

**FIGURE 3.6**   The mandible.

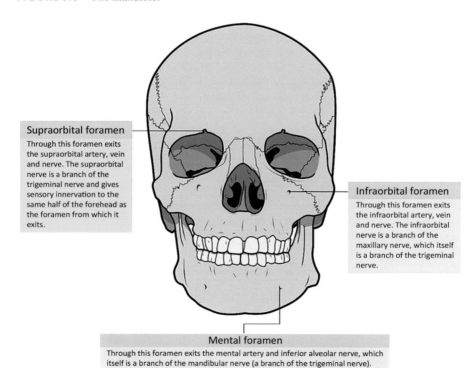

**Supraorbital foramen**

Through this foramen exits the supraorbital artery, vein and nerve. The supraorbital nerve is a branch of the trigeminal nerve and gives sensory innervation to the same half of the forehead as the foramen from which it exits.

**Infraorbital foramen**

Through this foramen exits the infraorbital artery, vein and nerve. The infraorbital nerve is a branch of the maxillary nerve, which itself is a branch of the trigeminal nerve.

**Mental foramen**

Through this foramen exits the mental artery and inferior alveolar nerve, which itself is a branch of the mandibular nerve (a branch of the trigeminal nerve).

**FIGURE 3.7**   Facial foramina.

## THE FACIAL NERVE

The facial nerve is the seventh cranial nerve and is responsible for controlling the movement of the muscles of facial expression and the sensation of taste in the anterior two-thirds of the tongue.

It is conceptually easiest to imagine the facial nerve as originating intracranially and terminating at the muscles which it innervates, therefore we shall start the description of the path of the facial nerve at the *facial nerve nucleus*, a cluster of neurons located at the anterolateral aspect of the *pontine tegmentum* within the dorsal pons. The upper aspect of this nucleus is responsible for the movement of the upper half of the face, whereas, rather unsurprisingly, the lower portion of the nucleus controls movement of the lower half of the face.

The facial nerve exits the pons at the level of the *pontomedullary junction* and projects through the cerebellopontine angle via the *cerebellopontine cistern* towards the internal auditory meatus within the *petrous temporal bone*. The internal auditory canal runs laterally through this bone for approximately 1 cm whilst it gradually narrows until it creates a fundus at its lateral boundary. The facial nerve enters the internal auditory canal via the anterosuperior quadrant and runs along this canal to the fundus, where it enters the *facial canal*. The facial canal is approximately 3 cm long and "Z"-shaped. Despite being small, it is divided into three sections, the *labrynthine*, *tympanic* and *mastoidal* segments. The facial nerve traverses the facial canal, giving off branches as it does so, such as the chorda tympani and the nerve to stapedius.

Once it has passed through the length of the facial canal, the facial nerve exits via the *stylomastoid foramen* which can be found in the inferior aspect of the petrosal temporal bone, between the base of the styloid and the mastoid process of the temporal bone. The facial nerve then travels between the *digastric* and *stylohyoid* muscles, giving off branches to innervate them as it does so, before entering the *parotid gland*. It then passes anteriorly through the gland before dividing into five terminal branches (Figure 3.8): *temporal, zygomatic, buccal, mandibular* and *cervical*.

### TEMPORAL BRANCH OF THE FACIAL NERVE

This is the most superior branch of the five extracranial branches of the facial nerve. It crosses the zygomatic arch and innervates the frontalis, orbicularis oculi and corrugator supercilii muscles.

### ZYGOMATIC BRANCH OF THE FACIAL NERVE

The zygomatic branch of the facial nerve traverses the body of the zygoma towards the lateral angle of the orbital rim. Along with the temporal branches of the facial nerve, it innervates the orbicularis oculi muscles.

### BUCCAL BRANCH OF THE FACIAL NERVE

The buccal branch progresses to subdivide into *superficial*, *deep* and *lower deep* branches as it travels anteriorly from the middle of the parotid gland, each with its own course and anatomical function:

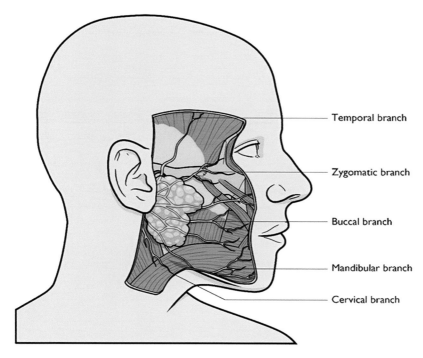

Temporal branch

Zygomatic branch

Buccal branch

Mandibular branch

Cervical branch

FIGURE 3.8    Branches of the facial nerve.

- Superficial branches pass between the skin and muscles of the face and innervate the procerus muscle.
- Deep branches innervate the zygomaticus and quadratus labii superioris muscles as they pass between them, as well as the intrinsic nasal muscles, such as nasalis.
- Lower deep branches innervate the buccinator and orbicularis oris muscles.

### MARGINAL MANDIBULAR BRANCH OF THE FACIAL NERVE

These branches traverse antero-inferiorly to the platysma and depressor anguli oris muscles before innervating the depressor anguli oris, depressor labii inferioris and mentalis muscles.

### CERVICAL BRANCH OF THE FACIAL NERVE

This branch is perhaps the least relevant branch of the facial nerve when considering cosmetics. As with the marginal mandibular branch, it runs antero-inferiorly to the platysma muscle before forming a series of branches across the suprahyoid region of the neck to innervate the digastric and stylohyoid muscles.

## THE TRIGEMINAL NERVE

The trigeminal nerve is the fifth cranial nerve and has the following sensory and motor functions:

- Sensory innervation to the skin, mucous membranes and sinuses of the face
- Motor function is derived solely from the *mandibular branch* of the trigeminal nerve which innervates the *muscles of mastication*, namely the masseter, temporalis, and medial and lateral pterygoid muscles

The origin of the trigeminal nerve can be appreciated as a confluence of three sensory nuclei: the *mesenteric nucleus* from the midbrain, the *principal sensory nucleus* of the pons and the *spinal nucleus* of the medulla oblongata. These three nuclei combine within the pons to create the trigeminal nerve root. The smaller motor nerve root also arises from the pons and can be found directly inferior to the trigeminal nerve root.

The sensory root of the trigeminal nerve extends anteriorly through *Meckel's cave*, where it forms the *trigeminal root ganglion* superior to the apex of the petrous temporal bone. The anterior and inferior aspects of this ganglion then divide further into three distinct divisions known as V1, V2 and V3 (Figure 3.9):

- The superior branch (V1) is the *ophthalmic* division
- The middle branch (V2) is the *maxillary* division
- The inferior branch (V3) is the *mandibular* division. It is worth noting that the motor nerve root which has been accompanying the inferior aspect of the sensory root offers fibres to this division

As the trigeminal root ganglion divides into these divisions each branch takes its own intra- and extracranial course to afford its own sensory and, in the case of the mandibular division, motor functions.

### Ophthalmic division of the trigeminal nerve

The ophthalmic (V1) division of the trigeminal nerve runs anteriorly from the trigeminal root ganglion, lateral to the cavernous sinus before exiting the cranium via the *superior orbital fissure*. Once it has travelled through this fissure, it further divides into three subdivisions: *frontal*, *lacrimal* and *nasociliary* which relay sensory information from the forehead, scalp, upper eyelid, nose (apart from nasal alar) and cornea.

### Maxillary division of the trigeminal nerve

The maxillary (V2) division originates in the middle of the trigeminal root ganglion and follows an almost identical intracranial path to the V1 division; however, it runs a slightly more inferior course, passing through the foramen rotundum before traversing the *pterygopalatine fossa*, posterior to the maxilla. Once the V2 segment has

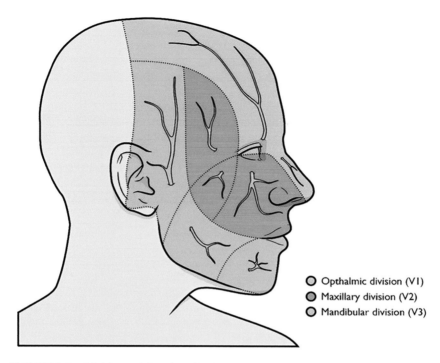

**FIGURE 3.9** Divisions of the trigeminal nerve.

travelled the length of the pterygopalatine fossa it turns superolaterally, entering the orbit via the *inferior orbital fissure*. It continues to pass along the floor of the orbit before arriving on the face via the *infraorbital foramen* of the maxilla, which is located inferiorly and slightly medial to the centre of the orbit.

The maxillary branch has the most complex anatomy of the three divisions of the trigeminal nerve, eventually dividing into 14 separate subdivisions. It is not necessary to know the names of all these subdivisions; however, you should be aware that its branches relay sensory information from the lower eyelid, cheeks, nasal alar, and the upper lip, teeth and palate.

### MANDIBULAR DIVISION OF THE TRIGEMINAL NERVE

The mandibular (V3) division of the trigeminal nerve is unique compared to the other branches in that it has both motor and sensory functions. It is the most inferior division and arises from the lower portion of the trigeminal root ganglion. Once it has branched from the ganglion, it travels anteriorly along the floor of Meckel's cave and through the *foramen ovale* of the *sphenoid bone* (posterolateral to the foramen rotundum). The nerve is then sandwiched between the *medial tensor muscle of the velum palatinium* and *lateral pterygoid* muscle as it continues to head anteriorly before dividing into a thin anterior and thick posterior trunk.

The thin anterior trunk offers motor function to the muscles of mastication as well as dividing into the *buccal branch* of the mandibular nerve, which gives sensory innervation to the buccal membranes of the cheek and second and third lower molars. The larger posterior trunk gives sensory innervation to the skin of the bottom lip, jaw, preauricular and temporal areas, anterior two-thirds of the tongue and the teeth of the lower jaw.

In the realms of cosmetics, arguably the most important branch of the mandibular nerve is the *mental nerve*, which branches from the *inferior alveolar nerve* (an inferior branch of the mandibular nerve) at the lower premolars. The mental nerve then runs anteriorly through the mandibular canal before exiting via the *mental foramen* allow for sensory innervation of the chin and lower lip. As previously discussed, the mental foramen is can be easily occluded during the augmentation of the chin with deeper fillers, resulting in potentially permanent damage to the distal mental nerve.

## FACIAL VASCULATURE

### THE FACIAL ARTERY

This artery is responsible for supplying the majority of oxygenated blood to the soft tissues of the face. It originates from the external carotid artery within the carotid triangle, deep to the ramus of the mandible. After branching from the external carotid artery, it travels anteriorly and wraps around the inferior aspect of the body of the mandible before coursing a tortuous path superiorly, past the corner of the mouth towards the cheek and nasal alar. The facial artery then continues to run along the lateral aspect of the nose to the medial commissure of the eye before it terminates as the *angular artery*.

As the facial artery courses superiorly, it gives off various branches to deliver oxygenated blood to the superficial structures of the face. Some of the more pertinent branches to cosmetics are the inferior and superior labial arteries, the lateral nasal branch, and the angular artery. The inferior and superior labial arteries supply the lower and upper lips, respectively. The inferior labial artery branches off at the angle of the mouth and passes horizontally in a medial direction between the orbicularis oris muscle and overlying mucous membranes of the lip. It is worth noting that it runs a very tortuous path, and therefore, it is almost impossible to ascertain its exact location through surface anatomy alone. Upon meeting the midline, the inferior labial artery anastomoses with the contralateral inferior labial artery. The superior labial artery, as its name suggests, offers arterial blood supply to the upper lip. It branches off slightly superiorly to the inferior labial artery and follows a similar, tortuous course horizontally along the superficial aspect of the orbicularis oris between it and the mucous membranes of the upper lip. As it heads medially it branches off into vessels which head superiorly to supply the nasal septum and tip of the nose (septal branch), as well as an alar branch which supplies the nasal alar.

The lateral nasal branch of the facial artery runs alongside the nasal bone and branches off into tiny vessels which anastomose with the alar and septal branches of the superior labial artery to give an increased blood supply to these areas, as well

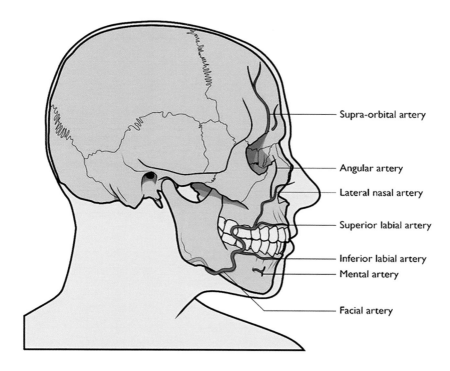

**FIGURE 3.10**   The facial artery and its branches.

as perforators to supply the skin overlying the bridge of the nose in conjunction with branches of the ophthalmic artery and infraorbital branches of the maxillary artery.

The angular artery is the termination of the facial artery as it heads superiorly and medially towards the medial commissure of the eye. It supplies arterial blood to the orbicularis oculi muscles as well as the lacrimal sac. See Figure 3.10.

### THE FACIAL VEIN

This vein is best understood by first appreciating its originating branches. The most distal supply of this vein arguably comes from the *superficial temporal vein*. This vein is which is situated on the lateral aspect of the top of the skull and forms a venous plexus with the *frontal vein* from the contralateral side of the skull. It proceeds to travel inferiorly along the anterior skull before joining the *frontal* and *superior orbital veins* which drain the forehead, eyelids and glabellar complex. Proximal to these anastomoses it is referred to as the *angular vein*, which then travels obliquely in an inferolateral direction on the lateral aspect of the nasal bone, draining tiny perforators from the skin overlying the nasal bridge before being joined by the vein of the nasal alar, otherwise known as the *nasal arch*. It is worth noting that the angular vein communicates with the *ophthalmic vein* and subsequently through these vessels blood can drain directly into the cavernous sinus, which can allow infections or

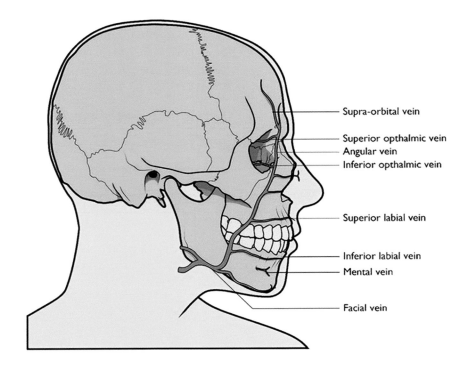

- Supra-orbital vein
- Superior opthalmic vein
- Angular vein
- Inferior opthalmic vein
- Superior labial vein
- Inferior labial vein
- Mental vein
- Facial vein

**FIGURE 3.11**   The facial vein and its tributaries.

emboli from the angular vein or its tributaries to easily cause complications such as intracerebral abscesses, infarction or encephalitis.

*The facial vein* is a direct communication of the angular vein which commences at the *root of the nose* (between the eyebrows). It is located inferiorly to the facial artery, yet its course is far straighter than its arterial companion. It travels inferolaterally to the zygomaticus major and minor muscles and along the anterior aspect of the masseter. As it passes inferiorly it gains tributaries from the *superior and inferior labial veins* which drain the upper and lower lips, respectively. It proceeds to traverse the body of the mandible before curving backwards deep to the *platysma* muscle. Once it has reached the platysma, the facial vein is joined by the anterior division of the *temporo-maxillary vein* to form the *common facial vein*, which itself drains into the *external jugular vein*. See Figure 3.11.

## FACIAL MUSCLES

The muscles of the face are one of the most fascinating and intricate systems one could ever imagine. They work in seamless conjunction with one another to allow us to perform all manner of complex tasks, including whistling, eating, drinking, smiling, frowning and many more. Cosmetic botulinum toxin administration will purposefully inhibit a person from utilising carefully selected areas of their face as they normally would to prevent the development and decrease the prominence

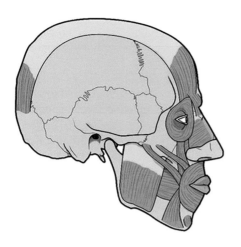 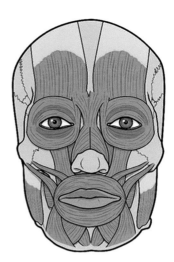

**FIGURE 3.12**  Muscles of the face.

of static lines and wrinkles. Due to the complexity of the facial muscular anatomy, it is all too easy to paralyse the wrong muscle groups, which may result in undesirable effects such as facial asymmetry and ptosis. Honing your knowledge of the facial muscular anatomy will not only make you a much more skilled practitioner but also give you the opportunity to proceed with treatments in the knowledge that your therapies are administered in as safe and effective a way as possible. See Figure 3.12.

## THE FOREHEAD

The muscles of the forehead primarily allow us to do two things: raise our eyebrows and frown. The forehead allows a person to quickly and succinctly express emotion to all around them, for example when surprised or annoyed. As we age our skin becomes less elastic and static lines commonly develop in areas of frequent, repeated motion as well as those exposed to the sun. The forehead is no exception to these rules and, therefore, is a commonplace for botulinum toxin treatment, with the intention of decreasing the prominence of dynamic wrinkles and preventing the formation of static lines in this area.

There are two main muscle groups responsible for forehead movement: the *frontalis* which raises the eyebrows, and the *procerus* and *corrugator supercilii* muscles which allow us to frown.

### FRONTALIS

The frontalis muscle is the primary elevator of the eyebrows, and it is a long flat muscle which runs across the anterior aspect of the frontal bone of your skull. One of the things which makes the frontalis muscle unique is that it has no bony attachments and, instead, attaches to the muscles surrounding it. The medial continuity of the frontalis muscle is the procerus; inferiorly, it is continuous with the corrugators and orbicularis oculi muscles and laterally with the orbicularis oculi and temporalis muscles (Figure 3.13).

Innervation of the frontalis muscle comes from temporal branches of the facial nerve, which arise from the facial nerve once it has exited the stylomastoid foramen. The temporal branches then track across the zygomatic arch and spread superiorly and laterally.

The arterial supply of the frontalis muscle comes from the supraorbital and supratrochlear arteries. The supraorbital artery is a branch of the ophthalmic artery,

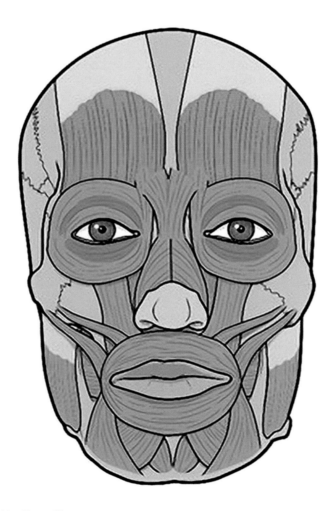

**FIGURE 3.13**   Frontalis.

which, in turn, is the first branch from the internal carotid artery distal to the cavernous sinus. The trochlear artery is itself a branch of the ophthalmic artery, its origin is within the orbit. We shan't dwell on intra-orbital anatomy too much, as it is not overly relevant for botulinum toxin nor dermal filler administration. You do need to be aware, however, that the supraorbital artery leaves the orbit and enters the soft tissues of the forehead via the *supraorbital notch*: a notch in the frontal bone just underneath the midpoint of the eyebrow, which you should be able to palpate with relative ease. It is imperative that you do not administer botulinum toxin or dermal filler in this region unless you have a very good reason for doing so, as you may accidentally inject it directly into the artery, potentially causing complications such as systemic spread of botulinum toxin, avascular necrosis, embolisation of filler or even pseudoaneurysm formation.

The frontalis muscle is drained by the supraorbital vein which runs inferiorly in the subcutaneous tissues anterior to the frontalis muscle. First, it gives off a branch which directly communicates with the superior ophthalmic vein before it dives into the supraorbital notch. The supraorbital vein then continues inferomedially into the orbit where it joins the frontal vein at the medial angle of the orbit to form the angular vein.

The reason why it is imperative to understand the venous drainage of the forehead in the context of dermal filler and botulinum toxin therapy is that the superior ophthalmic vein drains directly into the *cavernous sinus*, a collection of venous channels located between the meninges and endosteum of the temporal and sphenoid bones in a cavity called the lateral sella compartment, which can be found immediately lateral to the sella turcica, where the pituitary gland is located. Alongside the venous component, the internal carotid artery and oculomotor, trochlear, trigeminal and abducens nerves pass through the cavernous sinus.

The clinical significance of the cavernous sinus is that infection in the forehead, such as cellulitis secondary to botulinum toxin administration, may drain directly into the cavernous sinus via the superior ophthalmic vein. Due to the close proximity of the meninges to the cavernous sinus, this may mean that a person could develop a life-threatening meningitis were this to happen. Another potential cause of concern regarding treating regions drained by the superior orbital vein is embolisation of infection (such as in the setting of thrombophlebitis) or dermal filler products resulting in cavernous sinus thrombosis, which may result in life-threatening infection or permanent damage of the cranial nerves which pass through the sinus itself.

## PROCERUS

The procerus muscle is a pyramid-shaped muscle which arises from fascia over the lower portion of the nasal bone and the lateral nasal cartilage. It inserts into the skin between the eyebrows with superior fibres, attaching to the inferior border of the frontalis muscle. As you may be able to infer from its location, the procerus muscle is involved with pulling the eyebrows down and together, thus allowing a person to scowl. As an aside, the procerus also has a secondary function in flaring the nostrils. See Figure 3.14.

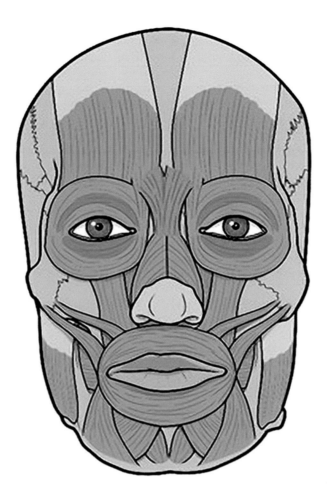

**FIGURE 3.14**   Procerus.

Superficial branches of the buccal branch of the facial nerve innervate the procerus muscles. The buccal branches come off from the facial nerve after it has exited the stylomastoid foramen and spread transversely to supply the muscles around the mouth and in the infraorbital region.

There is some contention as to the predominant artery supplying the procerus muscle, with some anatomists arguing it is supplied by branches of the facial artery tracking superiorly along the lateral aspect of the nasal bone, whereas others suggest that it is supplied by branches of the supraorbital ophthalmic artery, which you should be familiar with from the previous section on the frontalis muscle. The facial artery arises from the *external* carotid artery (the ophthalmic artery arises from the *internal* carotid artery) slightly superior to the lingual artery. After branching from the external carotid artery, the facial artery dips medially to the angle of the mandible before curving underneath it and heading superiorly along the mandibular ramus, branching off the superior and inferior labial arteries which supply the top and bottom lips respectively. The facial artery continues to take a tortuous path up the maxillary bone and then parallel to the nasal bone, heading superiorly until it terminates as the angular artery in the corner of the eye.

As with the frontalis muscle, the procerus is also drained by the supraorbital vein, and treatment of this region therefore confers the same risk of cavernous sinus thrombosis.

### CORRUGATOR SUPERCILII

The corrugator supercilii muscles (colloquially known as the corrugators) arise from the medial aspect of the supraorbital ridge (the superior bony border of the orbit) and their fibres extend superiorly between the orbicularis oculi muscles before attaching in the deep tissues immediately superior to the midline of the supraorbital ridge. Regarding the relevant local musculature, the corrugators can be found lateral to the procerus, inferior to the frontalis and superior to the orbicularis oculi muscles (Figure 3.15).

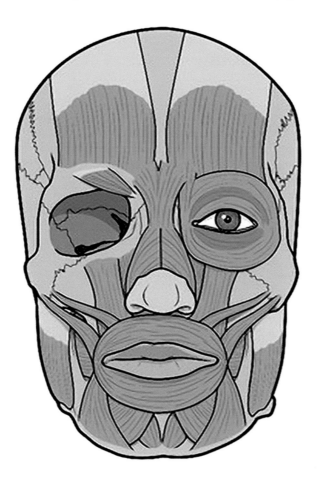

FIGURE 3.15    Corrugator supercilii.

The function of the corrugators is to allow a person to frown or squint by pulling the eyebrows medially and inferiorly. One potentially undesirable cosmetic side effect of this is the vertical lines created in doing so, and therefore, it is a common location for a person to request dermal fillers or botulinum toxin therapy.

The corrugators are innervated by the temporal branches of the facial nerve and their arterial supply comes from the ophthalmic artery, as described when we discussed the frontalis muscle. In some people, the lateral aspect of the corrugators also receives some of their arterial supply from branches of the superior temporal artery, which itself is a branch of the external carotid artery. The superficial temporal artery further has parietal and frontal branches. It is the frontal branches that are of interest to us regarding the arterial supply of the corrugator supercilii muscles. The parietal branches curve posteriorly and superiorly to join up with the posterior auricular and occipital arteries.

Finally, the venous drainage of the corrugators is the same as that of the procerus muscles, and the subsequently, treatment in this region carries the same risks regarding the cavernous sinus as when treating the procerus.

## THE CHEEKS AND MOUTH

### ORBICUARIS OCULI

The orbicularis oculi muscles can be found in a ring surrounding the anterior portion of the orbit and play a key role in closing the eyes. These muscles arise from the medial portion of the frontal and lacrimal bones and insert into the lateral palpebral raphe (a ligament on the lateral border of the eyelids). Arterial supply to the orbicularis oculi muscle is primarily from the ophthalmic artery as well as laterally from the zygomatico-orbital artery (a branch of the middle temporal artery) and medially from the angular artery, which itself is the terminal branch of the facial artery. The medial venous drainage of the orbicularis oculi muscles comes from the medial palpebral vein, which, in turn, drains into the angular and ophthalmic veins. Laterally, they are drained by the lateral temporal vein, which, in turn, drains into the superficial temporal vein (Figure 3.16).

The orbicularis oculi muscles are innervated by the temporal and zygomatic branches of the facial nerve.

The lateral borders of these muscles are commonly targeted for botulinum toxin treatment to address the wrinkles which form when smiling or squinting colloquially known as "crow's feet".

The importance of knowing the function and innervation of the orbicularis oculi muscles are twofold: first, bear in mind whilst consenting patients that only the lateral aspect of these muscles should be paralysed in botulinum toxin therapy. Due to the effects of the cheeks lifting when smiling or squinting and these underlying muscles not being treated, patients may expect small wrinkles inferior to this area after they have been treated. The second consideration when treating the orbicularis oculi muscles is in the case of accidental trauma to the temporal branches of the facial nerve, for instance in the case of cheek filler administration.

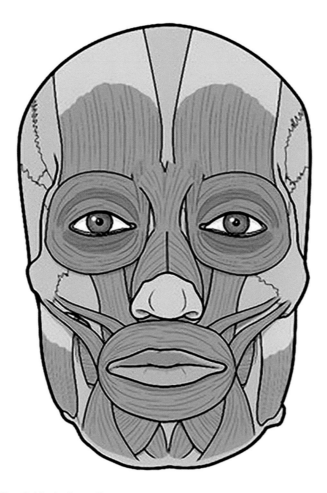

FIGURE 3.16   Orbicularis oculi.

Trauma to the temporal branches of the facial nerve may result in neuropraxia and subsequent paralysis of the orbicularis oculi and temporalis muscles. It therefore is prudent to keep this diagnosis in your mind should you have a patient with eyebrow droop who cannot close their eyelids on the same side as cheek augmentation.

### Zygomaticus major and minor

The zygomaticus muscles are muscles of facial expression and are found anterior the zygoma and maxillae. The zygomaticus major originates from the zygoma and attaches at the corner of the mouth. When it contracts, it pulls the corner of the mouth superiorly

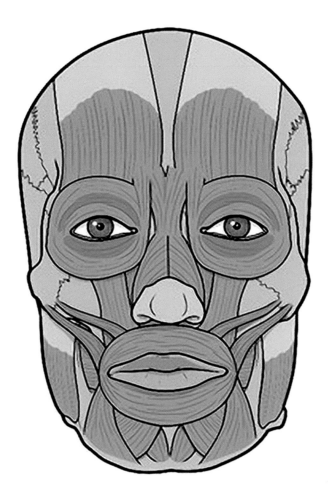

**FIGURE 3.17**   Zygomaticus major and minor.

and posteriorly to allow a person to smile. The zygomaticus minor is a slightly smaller muscle located superior and medial to the zygomaticus major. It, too, arises from the zygoma and is involved in smiling; however, this muscle inserts to the outer top lip and pulls the top lip superiorly, laterally and posteriorly, and aids the zygomaticus major in helping a person perform a smile. Both the zygomaticus muscles receive an arterial supply from the facial artery and are stimulated by the buccal and zygomatic branches of the facial nerve. The venous drainage of the zygomaticus muscles comes from the facial vein which drains into the internal jugular vein. See Figure 3.17.

## LEVATOR LABII SUPERIORIS

The levator labii superioris muscle is found on the medial cheek between the zygomaticus muscles and the nose. It is a broad muscle which originates on the

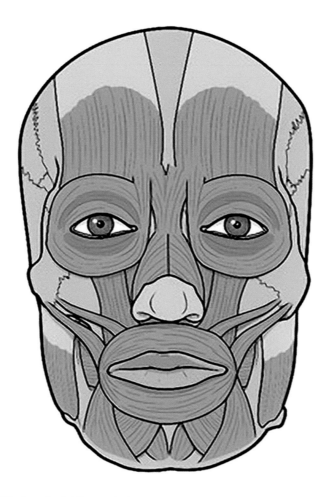

**FIGURE 3.18**    Levator labii superioris.

inferomedial aspect of the orbital rim and inserts on the top lip and nasal alar. It has two primary functions: One is to flare the nostrils, and the other is to raise the top lip. It is supplied arterially by the facial artery and drained by the facial vein. The nervous stimulation of the levator labii superioris comes from the buccal branches of the facial nerve. See Figure 3.18.

## ORBICULARIS ORIS

The orbicularis oris is one of the more complex muscles in the human body. Historically it was mislabelled as a sphincter and was presumed to be a simple circular muscle to allow the mouth to open and close. Recently it has been deemed to be actually a grid of four interweaving muscle sections with the involvement of facial muscles, such as the levator labii and buccinators, to allow for the puckering of the

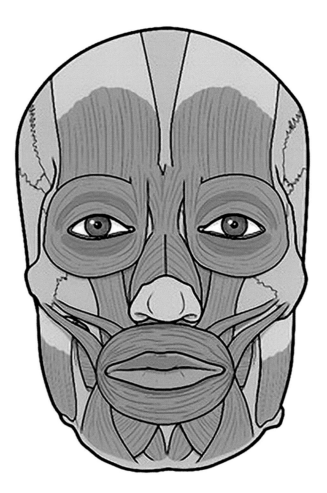

**FIGURE 3.19**   Orbicularis oris.

lips. These muscles are innervated by the buccinator branches of the facial nerve. See Figure 3.19.

The orbicularis oris is supplied arterially by the superior and inferior labial arteries and innervated by superficial branches of the facial nerve, which run through the lips between the muscle of the orbicularis oris and the submucosal layer. The labial arteries are easily damaged by direct trauma or occluded by dermal filler, causing resultant avascular necrosis; therefore, the utmost care is required when performing lip augmentation with dermal filler agents. The venous drainage is simple to remember as they accompany the relevant arteries and are unsurprisingly named the superior and inferior labial veins, which themselves drain into the facial vein and are vulnerable to trauma or occlusion from dermal fillers as well.

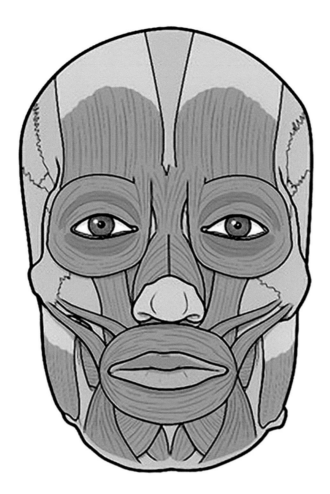

**FIGURE 3.20** Depressor anguli oris.

## DEPRESSOR ANGULI ORIS

This muscle can be located at the angle of the mouth. It arises from the mandibular tubercle and travels in a superomedial direction before inserting at the modiolus.

As its name suggests it, depresses the angles of the mouth, allowing it to become downturned. It is innervated by the mandibular branch of the facial nerve and receives its arterial supply from the inferior labial artery, with venous drainage via the inferior labial vein (Figure 3.20).

## MODIOLUS

The modiolus is an anastomosis of the buccinator, orbicularis oris, zygomaticus major, risorius, platysma and levator labii superioris. These muscles are all tightly

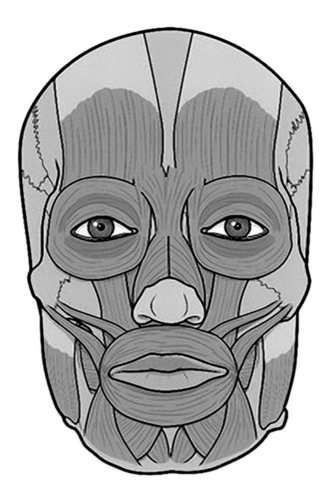

**FIGURE 3.21**   Modiolus.

bound together by interweaving strong fibrous tissues, which plays a crucial role in anchoring these muscles. They are innervated by the facial nerve and receives their blood supply from the facial artery. The venous drainage of the modiolus is via the facial vein (Figure 3.21).

## BUCCINATOR

The buccinator is one of the largest muscles of the cheek. It is a broad muscle which originates from the alveolar ridge of the maxilla, mandible and temporomandibular joint and inserts into the lateral fibres of the orbicularis oris. Its arterial supply comes from the buccinator artery, and it is innervated by buccal branches of the facial nerve (Figure 3.22).

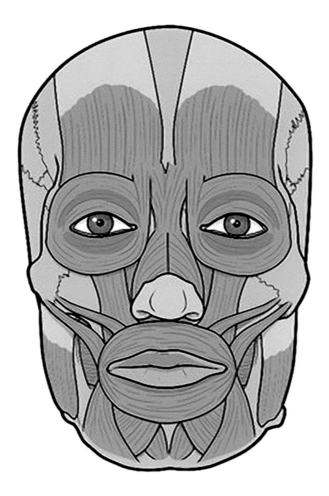

FIGURE 3.22   Buccinator.

## MASSETERS

The masseters are muscles of the cheek and lower jaw and are the primary muscles of mastication. They are important cosmetically as it is possible to make the face appear slimmer by administering botulinum toxin to the masseters. This treatment has, however, fallen out of favour due to the significant risk of localised (and permanent) osteoporosis of the mandible with subsequent fractures. They arise from the zygomatic and maxillary processes of the zygoma and insert on the coronoid process and lateral aspect of the mandibular ramus. Their arterial blood supply comes from the masseteric artery, which itself is a branch of the external carotid artery and passes over the mandibular notch, which is located between the coronoid process of the mandible and the temporomandibular joint. Unlike many other facial muscles,

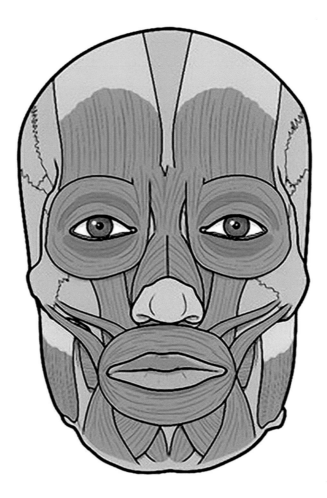

**FIGURE 3.23**   Masseters.

the masseters receive their nervous innervation from the trigeminal nerve or, more precisely, the V3 segment or mandibular nerve. See Figure 3.23.

### MENTALIS

The mentalis muscles are found as a pair located at the symphisis menti. They originate from the anterior mandible and insert into the chin. They function to wiggle the soft tissues anterior to the chin as well as allow pouting. They are therefore responsible for wrinkles demonstrated centrally under the bottom lip as well as on the chin. Its innervation is from the mandibular branches of the facial nerve, and it receives its arterial blood supply from the mental artery, which itself is a branch of the inferior alveolar which itself is borne from the maxillary artery. The maxillary

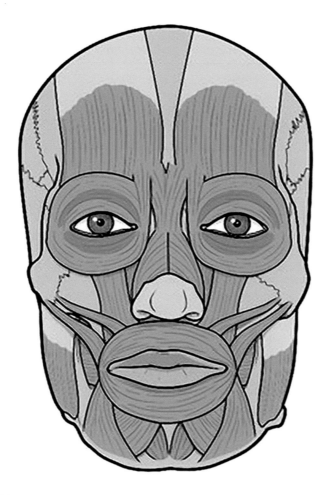

FIGURE 3.24    Mentalis.

artery emerges from the mental foramen, which can be found deep to the mentalis muscle. See Figure 3.24.

## FACIAL FAT PADS

Historically, the fat pads of the face were broadly divided into superficial and deep layers in relation to the previously described facial musculature, with the superficial fat pads sitting atop the facial muscles and the deep fat pads being found below them. Further distinction of the facial fat pads proved to be difficult, with somewhat arbitrary borders used to delineate them from one another. In 2007, however, seminal work by American plastic surgeons Drs Rohrich and Pessa utilised cadaveric studies to accurately, and reproducibly, discern the facial fat pads. In their research, they injected methylene blue into the facial fat pads of cadaveric specimens to ascertain their natural boundaries. These boundaries were composed of septae which separated the fat pads, allowing anatomists and surgeons to finally understand the true morphology of the fat pads of the face.

The fat pads of the face most relevant to aesthetic medicine are those within the midfacial region, as these contribute significantly to the outward signs of ageing, as will be discussed in Chapter 5. There are five superficial and fat pads of the midface, as shown in Table 3.1.

SUPERFICIAL FAT PADS OF THE MIDFACE

As detailed earlier, the superficial fat pads can be found superior to the facial muscles and are often easily palpated. The infraorbital fat pad can be found overlying the inferior orbital rim and the nasolabial fat pad courses inferolaterally along the nasolabial fold towards the corner of the mouth. Finally, the superficial cheek fat pads run in parallel course adjacent to one another, with the superficial medial cheek fat pad being located within the recess between the infraorbital and nasolabial fat pads and the middle and lateral cheek fat pads being found inferolateral to this, commonly overlying the zygomaticus and levator labii superioris muscles. Although the superficial fat pads of the face are not commonly targeted in aesthetic practice, they are often lifted when the deeper fat pads are augmented with dermal filler, therefore an appreciation of their anatomical location is useful, especially should they inadvertently become more prominent after treating the deeper fat pads or should they themselves be inadvertently treated with dermal filler. See Figure 3.25.

DEEP FAT PADS OF THE MIDFACE

The deep fat pads of the midface are commonly targeted with dermal fillers to restore volume loss secondary to ageing and mitigate the secondary findings due to this, such as overly prominent nasolabial folds. The term *dermal filler* is actually somewhat of a misnomer in such treatments, as the targeted region is supraperiosteal as opposed to within the dermal layer itself.

The medial and lateral suborbicularis oculi fat pads are found overlying the maxilla and zygoma of the inferior orbital rim before coursing superolaterally towards

---

**TABLE 3.1**
**Superficial and Deep Fat Pads of the Midface**

| Superficial Fat Pads | Deep Fat Pads |
| --- | --- |
| Infraorbital | Medial suborbicularis oculi |
| Superficial medial cheek | Lateral suborbicularis oculi |
| Middle medial cheek | Deep medial cheek |
| Lateral medial cheek | Deep lateral cheek |
| Nasolabial | Buccal |

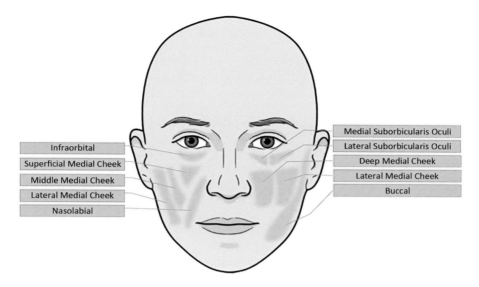

**FIGURE 3.25**   The deep and superficial fat pads of the midface.

the zygomatic arch. They are tightly adherent to the underlying periosteum and, unsurprisingly, are immediately deep to the orbicularis oculi muscles.

The deep medial and lateral cheek fat pads are located immediately superior to the maxilla, deep to the zygomaticus and levator labii muscles and the more anterior superficial and middle medial cheek fat pads. The deep medial fat pad often lies deep to the nasolabial fold, whereas the deep lateral fat pad is lateral to this, deep to the muscles and superior medial fat pad. When performing cheek augmentation, it is most commonly the deep medial and lateral cheek fat pads which are targeted to restore lost volume and "lift" the mid- and lower face.

Finally, the buccal fat pad is sited lateral to the deep lateral cheek fat pad and courses from the angle of the mandible, superiorly along the lateral maxilla and zygoma before terminating over the inferior temporal bone.

## LYMPHATIC DRAINAGE OF THE FACE

The lymphatics of the body are an adjunct to both the cardiovascular and immune systems, allowing the transport of lymph around the body. In this section, I discuss the lymphatic drainage of the face, head and neck, as well as its relevance when assessing your patients. Understanding the anatomy of the lymphatic drainage of the head and neck is crucial to minimising complications, identifying them when they occur, and addressing them promptly and accurately. It is worth bearing in mind that many lymph nodes have different synonyms and may be referred to by different names in different texts.

Although most of the fluid in blood is returned to the heart by blood vessels, a small portion remains as extracellular interstitial fluid. This fluid is high in white cells and drains into tiny, blind-ended, highly permeable lymph capillaries which collect fluid from surrounding tissues, carrying it into larger lymph vessels, which, in turn, drain into lymph nodes. Lymphatic vessels entering a lymph node are called *afferent lymph vessels*, and those leaving lymph nodes are called *efferent lymph vessels*. The lymphatic system has no central pump like the heart and instead relies on peristalsis of the lymph vessels themselves, as well as contraction of surrounding skeletal muscles. Anything which impairs lymphatic drainage, such as damage to lymph vessels or muscle paralysis, can cause an accumulation of tissue fluid, leading to lymphoedema and swelling. This can give a poor cosmetic result and may also leave patients at risk of infection.

Lymphatics are a crucial part of the immune system, as lymph nodes contain white blood cells waiting to identify and fight infection which travel along the lymphatic vessels to where they are needed. Lymph nodes may be become enlarged as a result of local infection in the area drained by the enlarged lymph nodes, otherwise known as *lymphadenopathy*. This is due to them becoming engorged by sequestered white blood cells actively challenging an infective pathogen. Therefore, knowledge of lymphatic drainage can help in diagnosing and localising infections. It is also worth remembering that lymph nodes are often the first site for cancer metastases, and this should be in the differential diagnosis for a patient with lymphadenopathy, especially if it is *painless*.

The lymph nodes of the head and neck aid drainage of lymph from the face, scalp and neck. They can be further divided into four main groups based on anatomical location, which form a ring extending from beneath the chin, around the jaw to the occiput.

### LYMPH NODES OF THE HEAD: FACIAL GROUP

The facial group of lymph nodes are found deep to the superficial muscles of facial expression and are responsible for lymph drainage of the face, eyelids, eyes, nose, and cheeks. With the exception of the *malar* lymph nodes, they all eventually drain into the *submandibular* lymph nodes. See Figure 3.26.

- *Infraorbital lymph nodes:* Often not present, a single node may be present near the nasolabial fold; afferent drainage is from the medial eyelids, canthus of the eye, and nose. Efferent drainage is to the buccinator and mandibular nodes.
- *Buccinator lymph nodes:* Found overlying the buccinator muscles near the angle of the mouth. Afferent drainage is from the lower eyelid, nose, cheek and temple. Efferent drainage to the mandibular and submandibular nodes.
- *Mandibular lymph nodes:* Lie over the mandible anterior to the border of the masseter muscle, adjacent to the anterior facial vein. Afferent drainage is from the cheeks and lower lips, as well as the infraorbital and buccinator lymph nodes. Efferent drainage is to the submandibular lymph nodes.
- *Malar lymph nodes:* Superficial to the zygomatic arch, afferent drainage is from the eyelids, lateral canthus of the eye and temple. Unlike the other facial nodes, the malar lymph nodes' efferent drainage is to the parotid lymph nodes.

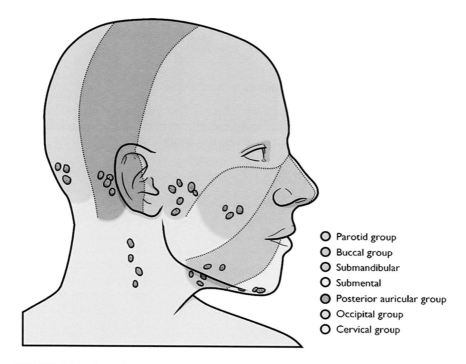

FIGURE 3.26   Lymph nodes of the head and neck.

## LYMPH NODES OF THE HEAD: PAROTID GROUP

The parotid group of lymph nodes lie over and within the parotid gland. They drain most of the scalp, temporal region, and ears as well as part of the nose, cheeks and eye. Some of these glands are found superficial to the parotid gland and others, deep within it.

- *Superficial extrafacial lymph nodes:* Located anterior to the tragus of the ear. Afferent drainage is from the forehead, temporal region of the scalp, the root of the nose and pinna.
- *Pre-auricular lymph nodes:* These sit anterior and deep to the tragus; afferent drainage is from the forehead, temporal region of the scalp, the root of the nose and pinna.
- *Infra-auricular lymph nodes:* Between the inferior border of the parotid and the anterior border of the sternocleidomastoid muscle, along the course of the external jugular vein. Afferent drainage from the posterior cheek, nose and upper eyelid.
- *Deep intraglandular lymph nodes:* Located within the parotid parenchyma, afferent drainage is from the forehead and temporal region of the scalp, lateral eyelid and lachrymal gland and the external and middle ear.

Efferent drainage of the parotid group is to the *deep cervical lymph nodes*, with the majority of these nodes following the internal jugular vein and draining to the *jugular lymph trunk*, a large lymph vessel in the neck.

### LYMPH NODES OF THE HEAD: MASTOID GROUP

- *Posterior auricular lymph nodes:* Located posterior to the ear. Afferent drainage is of the parietal and temporal regions of the scalp and posterior pinna. Drain efferently to the deep cervical lymph nodes.

### LYMPH NODES OF THE HEAD: OCCIPITAL GROUP

- *Occipital lymph nodes:* At the back of the head between the insertions of the sternocleidomastoid and trapezius muscles. Afferent drainage is from the occipital region of the scalp.

### LYMPH NODES OF THE NECK: CERVICAL LYMPH NODES

The neck contains some 300 lymph nodes, the two most important groups to know are the submental and submandibular nodes, to which a large proportion of lymphatics in the head drain:

- *Submental lymph nodes:* These are found under the chin between the two anterior bellies of the digastric muscles. Afferent drainage is from the lower lip, floor of the mouth and the tip of the tongue; afferent drainage is split between the submandibular lymph nodes and the deep cervical lymph nodes.
- *Submandibular lymph nodes:* These nodes are located beneath the mandible within the submandibular triangle. Their afferent drainage comes the cheeks, lateral nose, lips, gums and part of the tongue; it includes efferent drainage from the submental and many of the facial lymph nodes. Their efferent drainage is to the deep cervical lymph nodes.

Notch, C/EBP, MAPK, NF-κB, and KLF4. Failure for differentiation to occur properly can result in severe and potentially life-threatening diseases, such as Harlequin ichthyosis and dystrophic epidermolysis bullosa.

When keratinocytes reach the stratum corneum, they will differentiate no further, a stage known as *terminal differentiation*. Once they have terminally differentiated, these cells are known as *corneocytes*. Corneocytes are to all intents and purposes are dead cells, as during the process of terminal differentiation their nucleus, organelles and plasma membrane disintegrate. This disintegration process is driven by an influx of calcium, which, in turn, stimulates the release of tissue transglutaminases, which catalyse the cross-linking of proteins such as loricrin. These crosslinked proteins form a strong, waterproof sac to encase corneocytes. Whilst cross-linking is occurring, a lipid matrix is formed from lipids exuded from the terminally differentiating keratinocytes, acting as a glue to tightly bind these cells together. Once this process has finished, the terminally differentiated keratinocytes are stuck together in a strong, waterproof sheet. This structure is further strengthened by junctional proteins such as tight junctions and desmosomes between keratinocytes, which strongly adhere these cells to one another. By being both tightly bound and waterproof, the stratum corneum forms a barrier to protect deeper tissues from dehydration, poisonous chemicals and opportunistic pathogens. After approximately two weeks from the initial differentiation into a transit-amplifying cells, terminally differentiated keratinocytes are shed from the body via a process known as desquamation.

## METHODS OF SKIN HEALING AND THE INFLAMMATORY RESPONSE

Cosmetic procedures are almost universally traumatic to the skin. The delivery of treatments to the dermal or muscular layers inevitably involves a needle penetrating multiple tissue layers with subsequent microtraumas at each level. These superficial traumas are an accepted consequence of some of the more common cosmetic treatments, and although they are unlikely to confer any significant morbidity to your patient, knowledge of their physiology is important in becoming a safe practitioner. Understanding the effects of trauma at both a local and systemic level will prove invaluable in addressing any potential complications which may be directly caused by the treatment you have administered.

In principle, there are four individual processes which occur in response to local trauma:

- Haemostasis
- Inflammation
- Proliferation
- Remodelling

In essence, haemostasis is the process of blood clotting to prevent a sustained haemorrhage, inflammation is a response to clear out dead cells and potential pathogens, proliferation is the growth of new tissues and remodelling is the final stage, during which collagen is laid down and unnecessary cells undergo apoptosis, programmed cell death.

## HAEMOSTASIS

To administer botulinum toxin or dermal fillers the skin must be punctured with a needle, and whenever the skin is pierced, there is almost inevitably an element of bleeding due to inadvertent damage to microscopic blood vessels. The body counters this by initiating a haemostatic response which is triggered to stop fatal haemorrhage. In a healthy adult, haemostasis is fast and localised to the region which has sustained trauma. There are three primary mechanisms of haemostasis: *vasospasm*, *platelet plug formation* and *coagulation* which we shall explore in more detail within this section.

Vasospasm is the process of constriction of blood vessels by the smooth muscle which surrounds arteries and arterioles. This reduces blood loss in the local area for minutes to hours and is likely triggered by direct damage to smooth muscle, the release of chemokines from activated platelets and reflexes initiated by *nociceptors* (pain receptors). Adrenaline is a potent vasospastic agent and is released in response to painful stimuli, as well as being included within certain local anaesthetic agents to encourage vasospasm and decrease bleeding. One must be careful, however, when using adrenaline-containing local anaesthetic agents in close proximity to end arteries (such as the angular artery) as its vasospastic effects can cause localised tissue necrosis due to tissue hypoxia. In these regions, it is safest to avoid local anaesthetic solutions which contain adrenaline.

The second haemostatic process is platelet plug formation. Platelets are fascinating cells, laden with vesicles containing multiple chemicals important in haemostasis. These chemicals include adenosine diphosphate (ADP), adenosine triphosphate (ATP), calcium, serotonin, thromboxane A2, clotting factors and fibrin-stabilising factor – a chemical which is integral in strengthening and stabilising a blood clot. Platelets also contain platelet-derived growth factor (PDGF), a hormone which stimulates the proliferation of vascular endothelial cells, vascular smooth muscle and fibroblasts. These cell lines are crucial in the repair of the walls of blood vessels.

The first step in platelet plug formation is *platelet adhesion*, whereby platelets stick to parts of a damaged blood vessel, such as exposed collagen fibres of connective tissue on the inside of the damaged endothelial cells. Once platelets have stuck to the wall of a damaged blood vessel, the platelets become active and release their vesicular contents during the *platelet release reaction*. ADP is secreted to act as an energy source for activating nearby platelets, as well as thromboxane A2 and serotonin, which themselves are important in causing and maintaining vasoconstriction, decreasing the flow of blood to the damaged area and limiting further bleeding.

Along with its role in supplying energy to platelets, the release of ADP also causes nearby platelets to become sticky and adhere to the already-activated platelets during a process called *platelet aggregation*. This is the final step of forming a stable platelet plug, which is further stabilised by a mesh of fibrin threads formed during blood clotting. See Figure 4.2.

A platelet plug may be sufficient for sealing a small puncture; however, they are not strong enough to induce haemostasis in a larger wound. To ensure that we do not bleed to death, the body has another process in stopping bleeding: coagulation. Proteins known as *clotting factors* can be found within the plasma component of

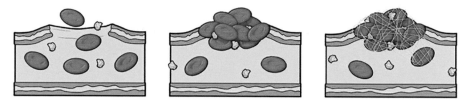

FIGURE 4.2   Platelet plug formation.

blood, and the majority of them are produced by the liver. Clotting factors induce coagulation via a series of enzyme-amplified events known as the clotting cascade. This cascade is made up of two interlinked pathways: the extrinsic and intrinsic clotting pathways (Figure 4.3).

CLOTTING FACTORS

Clotting factors are proteins which play a key role in regulating homeostasis and fibrin clot formation. The majority of these factors circulate the blood as precursors of proteolytic enzymes and are inactive unless activated by chemical mediators in the *intrinsic* or *extrinsic* clotting cascade. They are tightly regulated to ensure that

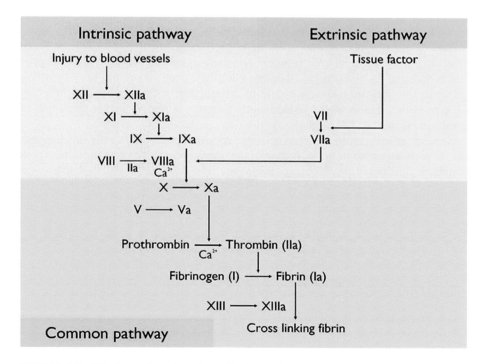

FIGURE 4.3   The intrinsic and extrinsic clotting pathways.

the blood does not clot too easily which may result in potentially fatal thromboses, as well as not taking too long to form a clot and putting a person at risk of exsanguination. The naming of clotting factors is somewhat complex, as the first four clotting factors identified retain their original names (fibrinogen, prothrombin, tissue factor, calcium) and the remaining eight are numbered with Roman numerals from V to XII. Almost all clotting factors are produced in the liver except factors III, IV and VIII. As nine of our clotting factors are produced by the liver, patients with liver failure are predisposed to longer bleeding times due to decreased production of these factors.

THE EXTRINSIC CLOTTING PATHWAY

This is a rapid sequence of events stimulated by a clotting factor III, also known as *tissue factor*. Tissue factor is secreted from cells outside the damaged blood vessel, hence why it is called the extrinsic pathway. Calcium secreted by platelets activates tissue factor, which, in turn, starts a chain of events which eventually results in activation of clotting factor X. Activated factor X binds with activated factor V (which also requires calcium for activation) to form an enzyme called prothrombinase, which we discuss in further detail later.

THE INTRINSIC CLOTTING PATHWAY

This pathway is slower than the extrinsic pathway and usually requires several minutes to become fully functional. It is initiated by activators which are either found within or are in direct contact with blood itself. Such mediators include collagen fibres exposed on the internal aspect of traumatised endothelial cells and phospholipids secreted from damaged platelets. Clotting factor XII is the initial clotting factor in the intrinsic pathway, and as in the extrinsic pathway, it results in a cascade of events ending with activated clotting factors X and V and the formation of prothrombinase.

Once prothrombinase has been activated by either pathway (usually this happens due to a combination of both), it cleaves the proenzyme prothrombin into activated thrombin. Thrombin then converts fibrinogen into its active, insoluble component: *fibrin*. As mentioned regarding platelet plug formation, fibrin forms a meshwork which stabilises the platelet plug. As fibrin fibres stabilise the clot, they also cause it to contract and pull the edges of the damaged vessel closer together and stopping the chances of further bleeding. Red and white blood cells are too large to fit through any residual gaps; however, plasma is sometimes able to seep through. This is why you may notice straw-coloured plasma overlying a healing wound before it becomes waterproof via a combination of clotting factors and the aforementioned platelet plug.

## INFLAMMATION

Despite being classified as the second phase of the healing process, the inflammatory process starts almost instantaneously alongside the previously described haemostatic mechanisms. The first step in this process is fluid leaving the damaged blood vessels, thus increasing the volume of the extracellular space. This provides a little compression to the damaged area to further decrease blood loss, as well as granting extra room for white blood cells to manoeuvre. Alongside its functions in the clotting cascade, thrombin also acts as a pro-inflammatory mediator by both attracting white blood cells to the area of trauma and increasing vascular permeability. By making capillaries more permeable, white blood cells can extravasate more easily into damaged tissues to aid the healing process. Blood vessels not only become more permeable in the inflammatory stage, but they also vasodilate to further allow the transport of immune cells to where they are needed most. This process is sustained by a medley of chemokines such as histamine, prostaglandins and leukotrienes. By increasing the blood flow to and from a damaged area, important inflammatory mediators and white blood cells necessary to process damaged cell components and fight infection can arrive more quickly, and toxic metabolites can be removed to the systemic circulation to be excreted. This process usually occurs approximately 10 minutes from the time of the initial injury. It is worth noting that the inflammatory phase contributes significantly to the sensation of pain due to injury due to swelling, tissue hypoxia and an altered pH caused by cell lysis.

White blood cells are attracted to the injured area by pro-inflammatory chemokines such as interleukin-1 to both fend off opportunistic infections and remove damaged cellular components. The first cells on the scene are *neutrophils*, and they are the main cell lineage present for the first two days or so. Their role is to directly challenge any potential sources of infection, be they skin commensals or microorganisms directly introduced via a penetrating injury. Whilst they are cleansing the affected area, they also release pro-inflammatory chemokines to attract macrophages and T cells to further modulate the local inflammatory process.

Macrophages are arguably the most important white blood cells in regulating the healing process. Their function is not only to phagocytose bacteria and cellular debris but also to secrete pro-inflammatory chemokines, enzymes and hormones which are crucial in the healing process. Examples of enzymes released by macrophages include elastases and collagenases which digest damaged proteins at the injured site to allow for remodelling to occur later. Their hormonal activity includes secreting PDGF which stimulates the production of fibroblasts and smooth muscle progenitor cells and vascular endothelial growth factor (VEGF) to attract endothelial cells to the wounded region to promote angiogenesis.

The final white blood cell lineage to approach a wounded area are T lymphocytes, which arrive approximately three days post-injury. Their function is to regulate the activity of collagenases to prevent accidental autolysis of healthy tissues and to commit pathogenic antibodies to memory to aid adaptive immunity, allowing prompt recognition and termination of these microbial species during future exposures.

## PROLIFERATION

Just as the inflammatory phase overlaps with the haemostatic phase, the proliferative phase overlaps with the inflammatory phase and usually occurs approximately three to five days after an injury has occurred.

The first step in the proliferative phase is *epithelialisation* – the construction of an epithelial covering over the external surface of a wound. This is important to keep water, toxic substances and pathogens out and to keep fluid *in* to create a warm, moist environment for wound healing to continue. Epidermal cells of either side of a wound will secrete collagenases which allow them to detach from the epidermal matrix and migrate towards the contralateral side of the wound. Upon arrival they stimulate plasmin production to degrade the clot formed during haemostasis, allowing for easier migration of epidermal cells. These cells are encouraged to adhere to the makeshift fibrin mesh over the wound to by fibronectin.

Whilst epithelial cells are busy covering the superior aspect of a wound, the *fibroplastic phase* is occurring underneath them. During this phase, hormones such as PDGF and fibroblast growth factor trigger fibroblast proliferation. Fibroblasts are cells which synthesise collagen and the extracellular matrix on which other cell lineages reside. By lying down the extracellular matrix, fibroblasts offer a scaffolding structure for migrating cells to travel across and adhere to.

The final stage of the proliferative phase is *angiogenesis*. Angiogenesis is the formation of new blood vessels and is vital in not only aiding healing but also sustaining life in the newly synthesised tissues. By creating and maintaining a new functioning blood supply, the necessary nutrients to support cellular proliferation can arrive expediently to where they are required, and the final degradation products can be removed. This process is stimulated in no small part by VEGF secreted by macrophages. As the healing process resolves, the need for hyperaemic tissues dissipates with this, causing the angiogenesis to cease.

## REMODELLING

The remodelling phase is also known as the *maturation* phase. This is the process in which your body alters both the macroscopic and microscopic appearance of a traumatised area and how a wound eventually begins to resemble its original tissues. Speed is of the essence in the haemostatic, inflammatory and proliferative stages of wound healing to stop dehydration, prevent infection and to stop tissue necrosis. In contrast to this, the remodelling phase is a much slower and more calculated process as hastiness is unnecessary once the vulnerable underlying tissues are protected and well vascularised, potentially taking months to reach completion.

Once a rough foundation has been laid down by these processes, collagens present are refined from a thick and disorganised type III collagen to a thinner and more neatly structured network of type I collagen. During this process, water is removed from the surrounding extracellular matrix to allow collagen fibres to lie closer together and therefore retract overlying scar tissue.

Collagen within the dermis and epidermis is naturally deposited along *tension lines* that run perpendicular to the underlying muscle fibres. These lines are of great significance regarding scarring, as wounds which are sustained parallel to tension lines heal with a far better cosmetic outcome than those which run across them. When a wound is healing, collagen is ideally laid down along tension lines to add biomechanical strength to the damaged tissues.

A combination of more tightly interwoven collagen fibres and reinforcement of tension lines strengthens scarred skin. It is worth noting, however, that despite the best attempts of the body to heal tissues in this way, scarred tissue is never stronger than the original epithelial layer.

## FACTORS AFFECTING WOUND HEALING

As previously discussed, wound healing is a complex, multifaceted process which relies on several physiological mechanisms occurring in conjunction with one another to ensure that traumatised tissues eventually resemble their original structure, function and appearance. The complexity of wound healing leaves it vulnerable to an array of factors that can cause disruption at any time from the creation of a wound to the completion of the remodelling phase.

The factors determining the success of wound healing can either be *local* or *systemic*; however, they are not mutually exclusive, and it is worth considering any and all elements which may affect the healing process when assessing and consenting your patient to prevent an unsatisfactory or unsafe outcome.

### FOREIGN BODIES AND INFECTION

The presence of a foreign body increases both the intensity and duration of the inflammatory phase of wound healing. Upregulated, prolonged proliferative and remodelling phases of wound healing result in potentially catastrophic consequences such as delayed healing, granuloma formation and deep-seated infections. It is crucial to adequately clean the area and maintain an aseptic, non-touch technique when performing any cosmetic procedures for this very reason. It is worth noting that the keratinocytes or hairs of your patient may be perceived by the patient's immune system as "foreign" if they are found in an unusual location, such as accidentally introducing a hair into the zygomaticus muscle of the cheek.

### EXCESS MOBILITY

In order for organised and therefore successful tissue remodelling to occur, limited movement is key, for example when putting a fractured leg in a cast. Restricting movement decreases the build-up of toxic metabolites and allows for the maintenance of a clot and the regulated deposition of collagen. In smaller wounds this is usually inconsequential as the degree of movement is limited, but bear this in mind when performing cosmetic treatments on the face as this is an area which is all but impossible to for a patient to keep still.

### BLOOD SUPPLY

The blood supply to and from a wounded area is crucial in delivering the necessary oxygen, white blood cells, and nutrients required for timely and effective healing and for removing toxic metabolites. Poorly perfused tissues do not heal well, and sometimes never heal at all. This is because oxygen, proteins and glucose are essential in affording damaged tissues the materials they require to heal, as well as preventing toxins from causing localised cell death and skin necrosis. This should always be a consideration of yours when treating a patient with known risk factors for vascular compromise, such as people who smoke or have diabetes mellitus.

## NUTRITION

Having a healthy diet and adequate systemic reserve is essential in wound healing. Malnourished patients have a dampened immune system, which in turn makes them more susceptible to wound infections and lessens the inflammatory response during wound healing, frequently prolonging this process. There are specific nutrients of importance in wound healing, such as protein, vitamin C, vitamin A and zinc. Protein and vitamin C are required for the proper formation and deposition of collagen, and subsequently, patients low in these nutrients often exhibit delayed wound healing and decreased tensile strength in healed tissues.

The evidence of the role of vitamin A in wound healing is at times vague; however, it is believed to be important in epithelial cell migration, proliferation and differentiation and therefore important in the epithelialisation phase of wound healing. Finally, zinc has been proved to accelerate wound healing, and patients who are deficient in it experience longer healing times than those who have a healthy, balanced diet.

## MEDICATION

Despite being prescribed with the best intentions at heart, medications can impair wound healing. Immunosuppressive medications such as glucocorticosteroids are particularly troublesome in impeding healing. Steroids suppress the immune system and therefore are used to treat inflammatory conditions such as rheumatoid arthritis and polymyalgia rheumatica. A decreased immune response will result in a weakened inflammatory phase of wound healing and impaired production of fibrous scar tissue. Having less fibrous tissue has negative implications for wound healing by both increasing the length of time taken for a wound to heal and decreasing the strength of newly deposited tissue.

# 5 The science of ageing

Ageing is a natural physiological process which affects every single cell in the body. One of the most common reasons people seek cosmetic therapies is to give the appearance of reversing (or at least slowing) the outward signs of ageing. True reversal of ageing is not something which, as of yet, can be achieved; however, in skilled hands, its outward effects can be masked. In this chapter, we discuss the hypotheses of how and why we age and ways in which the physical aspects of aging can be minimised.

## HYPOTHESES OF AGEING

Despite being a universal process, ageing is surprisingly poorly understood. This is likely due to the fact that every organism lives its life in a unique way, and therefore, there are almost limitless confounders for any data collected. It is also unclear as to *why* we age, a question which intimately blends science and philosophy; for example Longo *et al.* hypothesised that ageing and therefore *dying* is an altruistic process for the good of the species. By dying, there is less competition for resources, a decreased chance of the incubation and spread of disease, and tasks can be focused on the development and survival of younger individuals who may be able to offer greater support to their community, as well as passing on their valuable genetic material. Theories relating to the ageing process usually revolve around one of two key themes: *stochastic events* (random errors) and *programmed cell death*. In this chapter, we discuss a few of the better accepted theories of ageing; however, they should not be perceived to be occurring in isolation but more so as a series of concurrent, interlinked events which all, in one way or another, contribute to the ageing process.

### Somatic mutation theory of ageing

All cells within a multicellular organism (other than reproductive cell lines) are collectively known as *somatic cells*. Whenever a somatic cell divides, its DNA (Figure 5.1) is both transcribed and translated to create new DNA strands for its daughter cell. Each time the DNA is read, there is a chance of it not being copied *exactly* and a genetic mutation occurring, just as when one plays "Chinese Whispers": the more times a phrase is repeated, the higher the chance of accidental errors accruing in the final statement. Cells have mechanisms to rectify mutations in DNA:

- *Base Excision Repair:* Single nitrogenous bases are removed by an enzyme called AP endonuclease and the correct base is placed in their stead by DNA polymerase using the complementary strand as a template.
- *Nucleotide Excision Repair:* This mechanism is deployed by cells to repair longer segments of damaged DNA (up to 24 nucleotides in length) such as in ultraviolet-light damaged tissues from the use of sunbeds. When a damaged segment is identified, RNA polymerase will stall at the site of a lesion and

DOI: 10.1201/9781003198840-5

flag it up as damaged. This segment is removed by the enzyme *transcription factor II H* before DNA polymerase uses the complementary strand of DNA to synthesise the correct nucleotide sequence. Once this has occurred, the two strands are stuck back together by DNA ligase.

- *Mismatch Repair:* This process relates to nucleotide mismatches on newly synthesised DNA; however, the exact mechanism for this process is poorly understood. It is believed that newly synthesised DNA strands are monitored for mismatching, and should any erroneous sequences be detected, exonucleases remove the mismatched segment. Once this has occurred, the correct nucleotides are laid down by DNA polymerase and the strands stuck together by DNA ligase.

These DNA repair mechanisms work incredibly well at fending off potentially harmful mutations; however, there will inevitably be mutations which do not get repaired. This tiny margin for error is the crux of the somatic mutation theory: that as we get older, our somatic cells accumulate non-functioning or even pathological mutations of their DNA. Even if they pick up 99.9% of mutations, over the course of a lifetime a huge number of mutations will aggregate in all the somatic cells of our body. Evidence that DNA damage (and subsequent mutations) may be a key factor in accelerating ageing comes from cohort studies on patients with rare inherited DNA repair defects which demonstrate syndromes mimicking premature ageing. One such example is that of Werner syndrome, characterised by loss of the *WRN* gene which plays an important role in repairing damaged DNA via RecQ helicase and $3' \rightarrow 5'$ exonuclease activity. People with Werner syndrome cannot remove defunct nucleotide sequences from spontaneous mutations, and therefore, these mutations aggregate within cells over their lifetime. Due to the effects of accumulated and unrectified damaged DNA, patients with Werner syndrome will exhibit multiple signs of premature ageing, including thinning grey hair, atherosclerosis, diabetes mellitus, osteoporosis, cataracts and cardiovascular disease which we only usually expect to see in an older population.

When a cell accumulates a collection of genetic mutations which it cannot feasibly repair, it will undergo one of three changes:

1. It will choose to become irreversibly dormant and shut down all replicative function (a state known as *senescence*).
2. It will trigger apoptosis and destroy itself and subsequent its erroneous genetic material.
3. The cell will go rogue and undergo unregulated cell division. This is the initial event in cancer development.

Through senescence and apoptosis, our cells will try to do the noble thing to prevent damaged genetic material from being replicated and potentially causing our body harm by opting to never reproduce again either through cell suicide or becoming senescent. This strategy is employed to protect our body from genetic diseases such as cancer. As senescent cells do not contribute to homeostasis and apoptotic cells are dead, tissues with somatic mutations eventually have impaired function and contribute to age-related pathology, such as decreased renal function, grey hair and less buoyant skin.

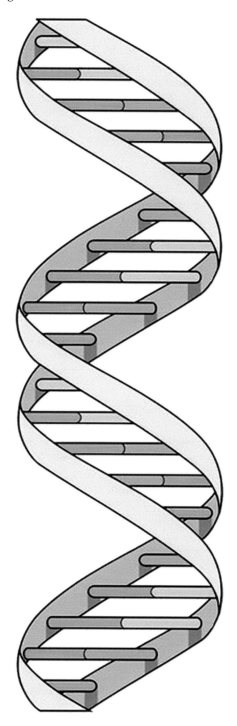

FIGURE 5.1 The DNA double helix.

## CROSS-LINKING THEORY OF AGEING

This theory of ageing was first suggested by Johan Bjorkstein in 1942, in which he hypothesised that an accumulation of cross-linked proteins damages cells, subsequently slowing down molecular processes and contributing to the ageing process. In essence, cross-linking is a chemical process which binds one polymer chain to another via covalent or ionic bonds, changing their shape and resulting in decreased functionality. One well-established process for cross-linking is *glycosylation*, during which glucose molecules are chemically bound to proteins, transforming them into advanced glycation end products, or AGEs. The added glucose molecules are naturally sticky and consequently adhere to other nearby proteins, altering their shape and creating a sticky gloop of defunct proteins. The accumulation of these AGEs over time contributes to the ageing process and age-related diseases, such as type II diabetes mellitus and atherosclerosis.

The body is inherently resourceful and tries, where able, to recycle defunct proteins to be metabolised and utilised elsewhere. Cross-linked proteins, however, cannot be digested by protease enzymes, and subsequently, these useless proteins will cluster within a cell. The build-up of non-functioning proteins in this manner results in a progressive impediment of normal cellular physiological functions. Regarding the skin, one key protein involved in cross-linking is collagen. Cross-linked collagen is far less elastic than it normally should be and is believed to be a significant cause of visible ageing, as it is far less elastic and retains less water, resulting in sagging of the skin.

## PROGRAMMED AGEING THEORY

The programmed ageing theory is actually three intertwined theories: *programmed longevity*, the *endocrine theory of ageing* and the *immunological theory of ageing*. These three theories are believed to run concurrently and support the utilitarian hypothesis that we age (and eventually die) to benefit the species as a whole. The programmed longevity theory suggests that throughout our lives from the moment of conception, various genes are turned on and off to cope with certain biological stresses. One piece of evidence for this theory is that within a species there is a relatively large range of individual lifespans; however, a maximum expected lifetime is relatively easy to predict. This contradicts some theories of ageing suggesting that as organisms age, they gradually decline, as some organisms (such as the fruit fly *Drosophila*) frequently die after a set life span despite displaying no overt signs of slowing down. It is suggested that having a stable genome as opposed to a wide genetic variability may indeed be a defining factor in the age somebody can hope to live to. It has been hypothesised that genes are turned on and off to survive biological and ecological stresses; however, most of us in the developed world are rarely severely physiologically stressed, with relatively easy access to food, shelter and medicine. One must consider ageing as therefore a genetic domino effect and that there is a clock ticking within each and every one of our cells with cell death being a pre-programmed end of a long chain of events throughout our lifetime.

The *endocrine theory of ageing* is beautifully intertwined with the programmed longevity theory; however, in this theory, it is suggested that hormones act as the pacemaker for ageing. One particular mechanism which has gained prominence in this field is that of insulin and insulin-like growth factor (IGF), otherwise known as the IIS pathway. The IIS pathway is an ancient hormonal regulatory system which is preserved in many vertebrates and invertebrates and has therefore been studied on animal models with a short life span, such as fruit flies and roundworms. Research suggests that decreased levels of insulin and IGF signalling will slow down the ageing process and even increase the life span of various multicellular organisms. This theory is still in its infancy, however, as it is difficult in larger mammals (such as humans) to determine the true effects of IIS signalling on ageing due to multiple confounders, long life span and molecular mimicry from hormones, such as growth hormone, which likely also plays an important role.

The final theory regarding programmed ageing is the *immunological theory of ageing*. Regrettably, our immune system peaks at puberty and progressively becomes less effective as we get older. This is partly because our body finds it harder to recognise antigens and the antibodies we produce become less potent. Due to having a physiologically dampened immune system, we find it harder to fight off infections and need to spend a greater amount of our metabolic reserve in doing so, hence why infections can be expected to affect the elderly more severely than healthy adults. A dampened immune system is also less able to identify and destroy cancerous cells and is likely a factor in the increased incidence of malignancies in older populations.

## WEAR-AND-TEAR THEORY OF AGEING

This is a well-established theory and one which makes perfect logical sense. If we were to use the analogy of a pair of shoes, the further you walk in them, the more they become worn, and if you never took them out of their shoebox, they would remain in pristine condition indefinitely. Our cells do not have the luxury of remaining in their box, and subsequently, they are continuously being "worn" by the complex metabolic processes occurring within. Under normal circumstances, cells have relatively effective repair mechanisms to ensure that no damage is done, but over time, these decrease in efficacy. If a vital and unreplaceable piece of cellular machinery becomes damaged, then our cells cannot combat the constant wear and tear they are subjected to and they will age and die. The likelihood of fatal damage to cellular components increases exponentially with time, as one would expect with our shoe analogy – the more frequently you use something, the more likely it is to break.

## REPLICATIVE SENESCENCE THEORY OF AGEING

Our cells divide at a predetermined rate and have a predetermined life span as discussed in the programmed ageing theory. The replicative senescence theory was suggested by the anatomist Dr Leonard Hayflick in 1961 after he noted that human foetal cells can divide 40–60 times before being able to replicate no more and becoming senescent. The number of cell divisions a cell can undertake has been named after him due to this work as the *Hayflick limit*.

The Hayflick Limit is determined in no small part by protective caps on the end of chromosomes called *telomeres*. Telomeres are repeating nucleotide sequences which function to shield the ends of chromosomes from accidental deletion or binding to adjacent chromosomes, and they themselves are protected by protein complexes, known as shelterin proteins, as well as the RNA, which itself encodes the telomere. By having these long base sequences at the ends of DNA strands, it means they can effectively act as a buffer to enzymes which may replicated the DNA erroneously. In vertebrates, the nucleotide sequences are AGGGTT with a complementary TCCCAA on the opposite DNA sequence. Overhanging this is a single-stranded sequence of TTAGGG nucleotides which repeat approximately 2,500 times in humans. At birth we have approximately 11,000 base pairs making up the telomere on the ends of our chromosomes, yet this decreases to approximately 4,000 in old age. The rate of decline in the length of a telomere is greater in men and is likely one of the many reasons men age faster and die younger than women.

Whenever our cells replicate, the telomere cap is reduced in length as DNA polymerase cannot restore the telomere nucleotide sequences. This is suggested to be one of the primary determinants of the Hayflick limit, as eventually the telomere will wear away to such an extent that the DNA itself is likely to become damaged. When telomere shortening reaches a critical level, DNA can no longer be replicated and the cell will cease to divide, becoming senescent. The aim of senescence is to prevent cells with aberrant DNA mutations from being able to replicate and passing on dangerous mutations. Despite this, research into human fibroblasts suggests the opposite may be true in certain circumstances. Senescent fibroblasts have been demonstrated to stimulate nearby precancerous skin cells to increase their rate of replication in older people and become malignant without affecting the replication rate of noncancerous cells. This may be reflective of an evolutionary trade-off, in that senescence may protect younger people from cancer by inadvertently predisposing malignancy in the elderly.

In certain cell lines (such as germ cells and stem cells), telomere length can be maintained by the function of the enzyme *telomerase*. Unlike DNA polymerase, telomerase *can* add repeating nucleotide sequences to the end of the telomere to mitigate the loss of length incurred by cell division. Telomerase is not produced within somatic cell lines, and therefore, its absence is contributory to the ageing process via replicative senescence.

When we relate the replicative senescence theory to cosmesis, one pertinent example is that of collagen. We know that collagen helps maintain the integrity and elasticity of the skin and is produced by skin cells such as fibroblasts. When skin cells become senescent, they lose the ability to produce collagen, and some even begin to produce collagenase which digests collagen. This is an important contributory factor in skin sagging and volume loss frequently reported by older patients.

## SYSTEMIC EFFECTS OF AGEING

When working in medical aesthetics, it is only too easy to simplify ageing as a process which only affects the *appearance* of a person, whereas actually it is a process involving every organ system within the body simultaneously. If this is not both appreciated and respected, then you may find yourself inadvertently causing harm to your patients.

As previously discussed, as we age, our cells inevitably lose the ability to undertake key metabolic processes and eventually apoptose, become senescent or undergo malignant transformation. We do not have the ability to notice the loss of functionality of individual cells, and instead, these changes are usually first noticed when an entire tissue or organ system is impaired. Changes can be described as either *age-dependent* or *age-related*. Age-dependent changes are those which can be perceived as due to normal ageing, whereas age-related changes are more likely to occur in an older person but are not necessarily directly linked to the ageing process *per se*.

In the realm of cosmetic treatments, *age-dependent* changes should be the crux of your assessment of an older patient. Decreased muscle, fat, and collagen will predispose to hollow-appearing cheeks, thinner lips or sagging skin. We must, however, always have in the back of our minds that older patients will have a physiologically weakened immune system and consequently are more susceptible to opportunistic skin infections post-treatment. Lower circulating levels of sex hormones such as oestrogen and testosterone can cause the skin to become drier due to decreased sebum production. As sebum is an oily substance secreted with the primary intention of keeping the skin hydrated, when less is produced it may predispose people to skin conditions such as atopic dermatitis.

Age-related changes are pathological changes which may affect every organ system as a person ages (Table 5.1). These changes include conditions such as cardiovascular disease, dementia, macular degeneration and malignancies associated

**TABLE 5.1**
**Age-Dependent Changes**

| System | Changes |
|---|---|
| Cardiovascular | Decreased maximum exercise response and tolerance |
| Gastrointestinal | Decreased gastric acidity |
| | Decreased colonic motility |
| | Weakened gastro-oesophageal junction |
| Hearing | Presbycusis (age-related hearing loss) |
| Hepatobiliary | Decreased liver mass |
| | Decreased blood flow |
| | Decreased metabolic rate |
| Immunity | Impaired recognition of antigens |
| | Decreased antibody function |
| Neurological | Impaired memory and concentration |
| | Impaired sleep due to insomnia and early morning waking |
| Overall body composition | Increased total body fat and decreased total body muscle and water |
| Renal | Decreased renal mass |
| | Decreased glomerular filtration rate |
| Respiratory | Mild obstructive pattern on lung function tests |
| | Mild increase in hypoxia |
| Reproduction (female) | Decreased oestrogen and progesterone with resultant vulval and breast atrophy |
| | Menopause |
| Reproduction (male) | Decreased testosterone production |
| | Prostatic hyperplasia |
| Skin | Decreased volume and synthesis of collagen |
| | Decreased skin elasticity and volume |
| Vision | Presbyopia (age-related visual loss) |

with increasing age (breast, colon and lung cancer, to name but a few). It is worth noting that the skin is an organ system too, and it also demonstrates significant age-related changes such as skin cancers, solar keratoses and atopic dermatitis. You must develop a keen eye for these changes when assessing a patient for treatment, as identifying a malignancy such as a basal cell carcinoma or malignant melanoma can save the life of your patient.

## FACTORS AFFECTING SKIN AGEING

The effectors of ageing in the skin can be broken down into *intrinsic* or *extrinsic* factors. Intrinsic factors are those which are specific to an individual, and primarily due to their genetic make-up, whereas extrinsic factors are usually down to a person's lifestyle, such as tobacco smoking and ultraviolet light exposure. One must have a good understanding of the plethora of intrinsic and extrinsic factors involved in ageing skin to be able to both treat and offer appropriate advice to your patients.

### INTRINSIC FACTORS OF AGEING ON THE SKIN

The various theories of ageing mentioned earlier in this chapter are all examples of *intrinsic ageing*. These are factors that an individual can do little about as they are dictated by their underlying genetics and physiological parameters. Despite the power of genetics, intrinsic ageing is actually a lesser determinant of ageing than extrinsic factors and is supposed to contribute to only 10% of the overall appearances of ageing demonstrated in the skin.

Intrinsic ageing within the skin has the same underlying molecular and cellular mechanisms as any other organ, closely resembling the effects of ageing seen in internal organs, with decreased cell turnover, decreased production of matrix proteins such as collagen, decreased extracellular fat deposition, and cell death or senescence. These changes result in a steady, generalised atrophy of the skin until we are about 50 years old, followed by a further, faster progressive deterioration. The cosmetic effects of intrinsic skin ageing are amplified and confounded by the more potent and preventable extrinsic factors of skin ageing.

### EXTRINSIC FACTORS OF AGEING ON THE SKIN

Extrinsic factors are external factors which contribute to the ageing process of skin. These factors can be minimised by lifestyle changes such as not smoking, eating a healthy diet, and not having excessive exposure to ultraviolet light.

### SUN DAMAGE

Skin damage due to ultraviolet light (otherwise known as *photoaging*) is the primary influencer in skin ageing. Its effects are generated from both natural exposure to the sun and, in a more dangerous recent trend: sunbeds. There are three main types of ultraviolet light: UVA, UVB and UVC. UVC light has the shortest wavelength and is dissipated within the ozone layer, therefore rendering it unlikely to cause any consequent skin damage. UVB light has an intermediate wavelength which can only penetrate to the level of the dermis, and it is believed to be responsible for the erythematous changes seen in sunburn. UVA light has the longest wavelength and, until recently, was not believed to be harmful to the skin as it requires *1,000* times the level of radiation of UVB light to cause sunburn. Recent evidence suggests, however, that UVA light *is* able to penetrate the skin to the dermal layer and may actually be responsible for the majority of chronic skin changes associated with photoaging.

Exposure of the skin to UVA and UVB light results in upregulation of matrix metalloproteinases within the dermis and epidermis. These enzymes further stimulate the production and release of collagenases by keratinocytes and fibroblasts which degrade collagen and elastin within the extracellular matrix. Decreased levels of collagen and elastin make the skin less buoyant and elastic than before it was sun-damaged. The skin responds by desperately trying to repair the damaged tissues; however, try as it might to re-create the original extracellular architecture, the reconstructed extracellular matrices are often irregular and poorly organised. Despite these flaws being on a microscopic level, over time and exacerbated by repeated exposures, these UV-induced defects in the skin eventually become visible to the naked eye in the form of wrinkles and sagging skin.

Both UVA and UVB light have the ability to damage our genetic material, not only contributing to the ageing process but also creating a very real risk of skin cancer. UVA is less energetic than UVB radiation and subsequently does not directly damage to our DNA but causes damage via reactive oxygen species known as *free radicals*. When UV light of sufficient energy strikes the mid- and lower dermis, oxygen is turned into the chemically unstable reactive oxygen species $O_2^-$. As molecules like to be in a stable state, superoxide ions attempt to stabilise themselves through a chain reaction which creates further highly energetic free radicals, such as hydroxyl radicals ($OH^-$), by stealing electrons from local molecules. Free radicals are known to cause damage in this way to lipids, proteins and DNA, damaging their molecular structure and consequently interfering with their function. Non-functioning proteins and lipids are degraded by cells causing disorganised architecture of connective tissues. Damaged DNA is more dangerous, as it can confer potentially cancerous mutations.

Free radical production is particularly important in the development of deep wrinkles through a process known as *solar elastosis*. Free radicals within the skin cause upregulation of the elastin promoter gene, which increases the production and storage of elastin within the outer dermal layer. Solar elastosis can be seen as a yellowish tinge to the skin with multiple deep crisscrossed wrinkles commonly demonstrated on the chest, neck and limbs. Further atrophic changes demonstrated in the skin are due to reactive oxygen species translocating glycosaminoglycans, such as hyaluronic acid within the dermal layer, and inadvertently modifying their primary disaccharide units. Glycosaminoglycans are usually found interspersed between collagen fibres, where their positive oncotic pressure draws in water to keep tissues hydrated. Free-radical damage to glycosaminoglycans means they are moved from collagen fibres in the dermis to elastic tissue in the superficial dermis. This movement of glycosaminoglycans means that collagen fibres become dehydrated and the skin loses fullness, further contributing to the appearance of older skin.

DNA has excellent photochemical properties and is, in fact, able to transform more than 99.9% of UVB photons into heat, thus allowing it to cause little or no harm. Regrettably, the remaining 0.1% of UVB photons are directly absorbed by strands of DNA in the skin, resulting in conversion of adjacent thymine base pairs into pyramidine dimers through the formation of new covalent bonds. Pyramidine dimerisation is not an isolated occurrence, with as many as 50–100 reactions occurring every single second when our skin is exposed to sunlight. As our cellular replication machinery has evolved to deal with sun-induced DNA damage; processes such as nucleotide excision repair are able to address pyramidine dimers within seconds of their formation. DNA strands containing pyramidine dimers which are not promptly repaired cannot be properly read by DNA polymerase, which may result in the arrest of cell replication or misreading during transcription and potential development of carcinogenic mutations. Pyramidine dimers can have devastating consequences if not recognised and managed effectively and are believed to be the key cause of the development of malignant melanoma in humans.

### TOBACCO SMOKE

The negative effects of tobacco on health are long documented and well understood, yet the effects of tobacco smoke on the skin are relatively poorly appreciated. It is believed that, similar to UV light exposure, tobacco smoke causes the upregulation of matrix metalloproteinases in the dermis and epidermis causing degradation of matrix proteins faster than they can be replenished. Smoking produces reactive oxygen species within the skin which, through almost identical mechanisms to the effects of UVA light, may cause elastosis within the dermal layer. Another important consideration of the effects of smoking on skin is that of tissue perfusion. Cigarette smoke induces a hypoxic insult to the body, and to mitigate against this, our peripheral vasculature vasoconstricts to ensure our visceral organs remain well oxygenated. A reduced blood flow means that tissues have less oxygen and fewer nutrients for respiration and metabolic processes, as well as a build-up of toxins in their local environment. These effects exacerbate one another in creating a hostile environment to cells and subsequently cause increased cellular stress, raising the likelihood of cell death or senescence. Chronic tobacco smoking causes atherosclerosis of blood vessels and may permanently reduce the blood flow to the skin with devastating effects such as poor wound healing, ulceration and tissue necrosis. A combination of matrix metalloproteinase upregulation, elastosis and chronic tissue hypoperfusion all contribute *en masse* to accelerate the ageing process.

## THE COSMETIC EFFECTS OF AGEING

We have the inherent ability to be able to make a snap judgement on whether we think somebody is "young" or "old" just by looking at them. Our perceptions of what constitutes an older or younger person change as we ourselves age; however, there are some key cosmetic features which we associate with increasing age, some more obvious than others. In cosmetic practice, you need to be able to objectively and to critically appraise a patient's face to allow you to slow the outward effects of age in a more targeted and effective manner.

Demas and Braun (2001) outlined some of the facial signs of ageing:

- Static lines on the forehead
- Drooping eyebrows, with a hooded appearance to the lateral upper lid
- A loss of cheek roundedness with deeper nasolabial
- Sagging neck wrinkles
- Decreased chin definition
- Perioral wrinkling and thinning of the lips
- Irregular skin pigmentation

These changes are important to identify by simply looking at your patient; however, it is useful to have an appreciation for what is going on at both a cellular and molecular level to be able to adequately counsel and treat your patients with the most suitable treatment.

## THINNER SKIN

The number of epidermal and subdermal layers remain unchanged throughout our lives; however, the thickness of the epidermis decreases as we age, especially in females and in sun-exposed areas such as the face and neck. The rate of loss of epidermal depth is approximately 0.64% per year, which may not sound like a lot but over the course of 30 years, it will result in a loss of almost *one-fifth* of the overall epidermal thickness. The dermis also decreases in thickness and vascularity as we become older, with fewer mast cells and fibroblasts present. Fewer numbers of these cells result in a weakened ability for the skin to mount an immune response as well as an impaired production of structural extracellular matrix proteins.

The subcutaneous fat deep to the dermis is also frequently thinner in older people with fat redistributed from the hands and face to the abdomen, waist and thighs – presumably to improve insulation and aid thermoregulation of the abdominal organs. A combination of thinner skin with less subcutaneous fat makes static wrinkles more apparent, increased prominence of nasolabial folds and volume loss around the mouth which may lead to a "sad" appearance.

## DECREASED ELASTICITY

As older skin contains fewer fibroblasts, it makes logical sense that it also has decreased production of hyaluronic acid, elastin and collagen fibres. As all three of these molecules are important in the buoyancy and elasticity of the skin, this decreased concentration results in the skin appearing less plump with impaired elastic recoil. Not only is less collagen produced, but it is also frequently more cross-linked and poorly organised, with resultant impaired strength, support and hydrophilic effects. The elastin produced in older skin is frequently photodamaged with consequent changes to their molecular structure, causing the skin to have decreased tensile strength and elastic recoil.

## Fat pad changes

Recent evidence suggests it is not simply sagging of the skin which contributes to the outward appearances of ageing on the face, but hypotheses have also arisen which suggest that changes in the facial fat pads are of importance in this regard. There are two main theories involving the facial fat pads: the older gravitational ptosis theory and volumetric deflation. These theories are unlikely to represent isolated events and are far more likely to be due to coexisting age-related physiological changes.

Gravitational ptosis relies on the supposition that tiny ligaments adhere the facial fat pads to the underlying bones of the face. As we age, these ligaments become weaker due to repeated movements of the adjacent facial musculature. These weaker ligaments are less able to support the facial fat pads against the pull of gravity as we age, resulting in a lower resting position of the facial fat pads in older persons when compared to a younger population. These findings contribute to a "sagging" appearance of the face as we age, with far more prominent folds between fat pads, for example within the nasolabial region.

Volumetric depletion is a newer concept when considering the effects of fat pads in the ageing face. Research by Lambros *et al.* in 2007 demonstrated that anatomical landmarks on the face, such as moles or the lid–cheek junction remained stable when comparing clinical photographs in a long-term follow-up study ranging from 10–56 years. They continued to hypothesise that were age-related changes purely gravitational, then these landmarks should surely descend inferiorly with the sagging skin. Their research further suggests that the underlying fibrous network of the face is relatively stable, and therefore, another cause for age-related changes in the face may be present, namely a loss of volume within the facial fat pads as opposed to simply an inferior migration. This theory is supported by evidence that administering deep dermal fillers in the cheeks does mitigate the outward appearances of ageing by simply adding volume.

Further studies suggest that there may be a predictable, chronological order in which facial fat pads atrophy, allowing for planned and targeted treatments to address these changes. It is believed the periocular fat pads demonstrate atrophy first, followed by the buccal, nasolabial, and finally deep cheek fat pads. These concepts lend themselves not only to diagnosis and assessment, but also for targeted and natural-looking treatments. Skilled practitioners can target the fat pads which are likely to be involved based on the pattern of atrophy and proceed accordingly to rectify changes due to volume loss or ligamentous laxity.

One final interesting observation regarding the facial fat pads and ageing is regional variation in the older face. Research suggests that the deep fat pads atrophy as we age, whereas the superficial fat pads hypertrophy. When considering an older face, stereotypically one can expect to see more prominent "bags" under the eyes and heavy jowls when compared to a younger person. This may be due to the simultaneous effects of atrophy and gravitational descent of the deep fat pads and the more superficial fat pads becoming more prominent. The reason this occurs is as of yet unclear; however, it is believed to be due to underlying metabolic changes associated with ageing.

Although the previously discussed age-related changes can be addressed with the use of deep fillers to lift the atrophic or inferiorly descending fat to decrease the outward signs of ageing, the best results arise from a surgical facelift or autologous

treatments are more extreme than others, and all offer their own particular risks and benefits. It is important to have an appreciation of some of the more common treatments so you can accurately advise your patients on a suitable therapy to address any age-related skin changes they wish to have addressed. One important aspect of the consent process is informing your patients of all available options. Should you believe a particular treatment you do not perform (such as a surgical facelift) would be the best treatment for your patient, then you should advise them accordingly. You are both legally and ethically bound to advise your patients to the best course of action in concordance with the most up-to-date evidence.

## DERMAL FILLERS

Dermal fillers are a versatile anti-ageing treatment and can be used to restore lost volume, hydrate tissues and upregulate fibroblast activity. Commonly treated areas include marionette lines, nasolabial folds, cheeks, lips and perioral lines as these frequently exhibit age-related volume loss. Dermal fillers frequently last for 6–12 months and usually have a small period of swelling or bruising for a few days post-treatment. They are widely regarded as the gold-standard non-surgical treatment for age-related changes secondary to volume loss.

## BOTULINUM TOXIN

Wrinkles can be either *dynamic* (present only on movement) or *static* (present during both movement and at rest). Botulinum toxin is a potent paralytic agent and should perhaps be classified as a primary preventative measure as it has little effect once static lines have formed. The effects of botulinum toxin last for approximately three to four months when a patient first starts treatment; however, it is not unreasonable to expect results to last longer due to muscular atrophy after subsequent treatments. This treatment should only be considered as an anti-ageing treatment for the forehead, glabellar complex and lateral orbicularis oculi muscles.

## PLATELET-RICH PLASMA

This is an autologous treatment with the patient's own blood being taken and centrifuged, separating erythrocytes from high platelet concentration plasma. The erythrocytes are discarded, and the plasma is reintroduced into the patient's skin. The evidence to suggest its efficacy is somewhat weak; however, it is gaining traction as a popular treatment to rejuvenate skin. The rationale behind platelet-rich plasma (PRP) is that growth factors such as platelet-derived growth factor and tissue growth factor are secreted from the α-granules of concentrated platelets once activated by aggregation inducers as discussed in the section on haemostasis. It has been demonstrated in vitro that PRP treatment may increase collagen synthesis and other matrix components through fibroblast activation. The increased collagen formation and fibroblast activity are believed to restore volume, hydration and elasticity to the skin.

## CHEMICAL PEELS

Chemical peels are believed to work by initiating the repair mechanisms of the skin due to transient inflammation secondary to epidermolysis and, if deep, inflammation of the dermis itself. The peels can be broken down into three categories depending on the level of penetration (Table 5.2), which, in turn, depend on the substance used (and concentration), pH of the solution and the length of time the peel remains in contact with the skin.

### TABLE 5.2
### Overview of Chemical Peels

| Classification | Chemical Components | Depth Reached |
| --- | --- | --- |
| Superficial | α/β-lipohyodroxy acids (HA); trichloroacetic acid (TCA) <30% | Stratum basale |
| Middle | TCA 30–50% | Upper reticular dermis |
| Deep | TCA >50%; Phenol | Lower reticular dermis |

Chemical peels have been shown to increase collagen, water and glycosaminoglycan deposition within the skin once the initial effects have settled, with subsequent improvements in both skin elasticity and wrinkle visibility. It is worth bearing in mind that these procedures have a significant risk attached, which increases with deeper peels. Common complications include opportunistic infections (especially secondary to herpesvirus), hyperpigmentation and solar lentigines. There is a significant recovery period after chemical peels, and this is unsurprisingly longer with deeper peels. Despite the risks, chemical peels do frequently offer significant positive results for patients with extensive age-related skin changes.

## LASER, INTENSE PULSED LIGHT AND RADIOFREQUENCY SKIN REJUVENATION

These therapies are frequently carried out by one of three methods: intense pulsed light (IPL), laser, or radiofrequencies. The overall mechanism of action of all three is similar; with an aim to cause selective, heat-induced damage to dermal collagen which in turn stimulates reactive collagen synthesis. These treatments are frequently deployed in treating photoaged skin and can be broken down into one of two categories (Table 5.3).

### TABLE 5.3
### Foci of Treatment of Photoaged Skin

| Type | Focus of Treatment |
| --- | --- |
| I | Ectatic vessels, erythema, irregular pigmentation, pilosebaceous changes |
| II | Improvement of dermal and subcutaneous cellular activity |

Evidence suggests that photoaged skin treated with IPL exhibits increased fibroblast numbers and new collagen formation in both the papillary and reticular dermis as well as decreased solar elastosis. IPL has been demonstrated to confer significant benefit for type I changes secondary to photodamage, with fibroblast stimulation and subsequent neocollagenesis and elastin formation in treated areas.

Laser resurfacing of ageing skin confers a multitude of rejuvenating effects, including epidermal ablation, collagen shrinkage and stimulation of neocollagenesis, regeneration of intracellular organelles, and an increase in the number of intercellular attachments. An accumulation of these events results in tighter, firmer skin. It is worth noting, however, that deeper laser treatments confer a longer recovery period and a greater risk of complications such as infection, persistent erythema and aberrant skin pigmentation. Recently there have been developments with fractionated $CO_2$, erbium glass or erbium-YAG (yttrium aluminium garnet) lasers. These lasers create highly controlled, microthermal areas within the dermis, stimulating wound healing, dermal remodelling and re-epithelialisation with a shorter recovery period and fewer side effects than traditional laser therapy.

Monopolar radiofrequency (RF) probes induce immediate skin tightening and collagen contraction through creation of an electric current conducted through the skin to the subcutaneous fat. The path of this current generates heat due to electrical resistance, which, in turn, results partial collagen denaturation followed by neocollagenesis and skin tightening. The skin-tightening effect is further precipitated by the inflammatory phase of wound healing. RF treatments have demonstrated good outcomes in the treatment of wrinkles, brow-lifts and addressing acne scars. Similar to laser therapy, RF treatments have a significant downtime of many weeks and confer a comparable complication profile.

## PHYSIOLOGY OF AGEING: RECAP

There are multiple theories surrounding the process of ageing, including the following:

- Somatic mutation theory
  - As cells replicate, errors in DNA accumulate with each successive replication cycle. Eventually the aggregate effects of these errors will result in the cell becoming senescent, apoptosing or potentially undergoing malignant transformation.
- Cross-linking theory
  - Accumulatios of cross-linked proteins damages cells, inhibiting molecular processes resulting in decreased cellular function and age-related diseases.
- Programmed ageing theory
  - Our cells, and therefore ourselves as a whole, have a finite life span which is regulated by genetic, hormonal and immunological factors.
- Wear-and-tear theory
  - Continuous metabolic processes eventually damage cellular machinery beyond repair, thus rendering them ineffective and contributing to decreased biological function as we age.

- Replicative senescence theory:
  - Cells can only divide a certain number of times (Hayflick limit) before they become senescent and cease to function. This is believed to decrease the chances of harmful mutations being passed on and cells becoming cancerous.

Factors which affect skin ageing in particular can be either *intrinsic* or *extrinsic*. Extrinsic factors contribute to almost 90% of the visible effects of skin ageing. Intrinsic factors are those which are specific to a patient, such as their genetic make-up, ethnicity and sex, whereas extrinsic factors are associated with lifestyle, such as sun exposure, tobacco smoking, and diet.

Certain physiological changes are associated with ageing of the skin:

- Thinner skin
- Decreased skin elasticity
- Atrophy and sagging of facial fat pads
- Dry skin
- Irregular skin pigmentation

Ageing cannot be prevented, but the cosmetic effects of it can be slowed by the following:

- Avoiding excess UV light
- Maintaining adequate skin hydration (orally or through emollients)
- Eating a healthy, balanced diet
- Using topical anti-ageing serums such as retinol

Cosmetic practitioners can lessen the outward effects of skin ageing through many treatments:

- Botulinum toxin
- Dermal fillers
- PRP
- Chemical peels
- Laser therapy
- Intermittent PLT
- RF treatment

Each treatment affords its own benefits and risks and therefore should be decided in conjunction with the patient's desired outcomes based on your clinical assessment of the primary causes of their cosmetic signs of ageing.

# 6 Patient assessment

Assessing your patients will be one of the most important phases of any cosmetic treatment. Alongside taking a detailed history from your patient, you will also need to understand the social and cultural approaches to beauty influencing treatment choices. It is important to be aware of what people perceive as beautiful and how your treatments can, and perhaps more important *cannot*, help them achieve their goals. You must not only assess your patient on a physical and psychological level but also have a good understanding of common skin diseases, as what a patient may perceive as an unsightly blemish may actually represent a far more sinister pathology. Having a keen eye for pathological lesions will allow you to direct your patient to the relevant medical experts and potentially save their life.

## APPROACHES TO BEAUTY

In 1757, the philosopher David Hume suggested that *beauty is in the eye of the beholder* and that we all have our own interpretation of what constitutes true beauty. It is undoubtedly true that each of us as individuals have our own opinions of what we find attractive in another, and recent studies suggest that beauty is anything but simple. Evidence suggests that we all have our own penchant towards certain traits we find attractive, yet this seems to revolve around a deep-seated norm which is almost ubiquitous across different cultures. One particularly strong argument which deviates from beauty being primarily a culturally driven phenomenon is that babies will spend more time looking at attractive faces than less attractive ones. Doing this at such a young age suggests that perceptions of beauty may be instinctive instead of driven by the views of those around us.

Further research indicates that an amalgamation of faces is seen as more beautiful than individual headshots. In 1990, Langois and Rogmann took a series of photos of individuals under similar lighting with comparable facial expressions before creating composite faces composed of 4, 16 or 32 individual headshots. They discovered that their study subjects found faces more desirable the more they had been averaged out, with the 32 amalgamations being deemed both the most attractive male and female face. This phenomenon may be due to the composite faces having blemishes diluted by successive layering or that averaging faces creates a sensation of familiarity in study subjects. Perhaps a more deep-seated and genetic reason for our predilection to "average" faces may be that as they lie closer to an expected norm that we subconsciously decide they are less likely to carry potentially undesirable genetic mutations.

It is far too simplistic to presume that averageness equates to beauty; if not, everybody would find it highly complementary to be labelled a "Plain Jane". Many of the world's most beautiful people have what one may consider striking features which set them apart from the rest of the population. Further studies on the back of Langois and Rogmann's work found out that composites of people regarded as *beautiful* were

DOI: 10.1201/9781003198840-6

deemed more desirable than composites of average faces. Another argument against the averageness hypothesis is that many of us subconsciously perceive symmetry as a beautiful trait. As an "average" face may have several asymmetries within it on close inspection, this would go against averageness itself being desirable. The view of symmetry as beautiful is due to the ancient instinct to have genetically strong and capable offspring. During embryogenesis, genes which determine the development of the two halves of the body are activated and deactivated almost simultaneously. Deviation by mere microseconds during this process will result in facial asymmetry. As it is our genes which dictate the accuracy of the timing of these events, we subconsciously recognise symmetrical faces as a reflection of a stable genome, which, in itself, is a desirable reproductive trait.

Features reflective of genetics and reproductive capabilities have been deemed as attractive for millennia. In females, this is perceived as having a youthful appearance, presumably due to a biological awareness of the reproductive difficulties frequently experienced by women approaching menopause. Research suggests that features deemed attractive in women include large eyes, a petite chin and nose, clear skin, a wide smile and large lips, which when combined suggest both youthfulness and sexual maturity. It is quite fascinating to think that cosmetic treatments are commonly requested to create this look that *Homo sapiens* have found desirable for hundreds of thousands of years.

There has been significantly less research into the science behind male attractiveness to perceived attractive features in females. Male faces which women find attractive seem to not only be related to reproductive capabilities and genetics but also an instinctive perception of a good father to their offspring. One of the key factors which give men a "manly" appearance is exposure to testosterone, which, amongst other features, stimulates muscle, bone and hair growth. Many species exhibit testosterone levels in different ways; however, in humans one easily noticeable feature is jaw width; men with higher testosterone levels usually have larger jaws than those with lower levels.

You may be confused as to how the jaw size of a male reflects both genetic stability and fatherhood, yet the logic behind this is relatively easily explained. First, testosterone acts as an immunosuppressant and subsequently people with higher circulating levels of testosterone effectively have a dampened immune system compared to those with less testosterone. The genetic significance of testosterone-induced immunosuppression is that those with high circulating levels are more susceptible to opportunistic infection and logically should spend a lot of time suffering with infectious diseases. Should a man reach adulthood in good health despite exhibiting the phenotype of a person exposed to high levels of testosterone, then this suggests that their immune system (and therefore genetic make-up) is strong enough to compensate for this physiological disadvantage. Being able to spot a potential mate with a good genetic composition by simply assessing their jaw size allows females to potentially choose a father to their offspring who will pass on a stable genome. As half of our genetic material comes from our father and half from our mother, making an educated guess towards a partner with strong genetic competence gives offspring a better chance of thriving. The second factor in perceived male attractiveness ties in with testosterone expression and varies with a female's menstrual cycle. Evidence suggests that at the time of ovulation, women will frequently select a male face with anatomy reflecting testosterone exposure as more attractive, whereas the rest of the time, many exhibit preference for softer, more classically feminine characteristics. Attraction towards a more masculine face during ovulation may tie in for a subconscious appreciation of a male's genome, whereas the softer features preferred at other points may be an ancient method of avoiding overly aggressive partners who could potentially jeopardise the safety of a woman and her children.

## ASSESSING YOUR PATIENT FOR TREATMENT

There should be five key questions you should answer when assessing your patient for any cosmetic treatment:

1. Do you understand your patient's desired outcome?
2. Does the patient have the capacity to consent to treatment?
3. Do they have the appropriate anatomy to create this outcome?
4. Is the patient free of any contraindications to treatment?
5. Do you have the ability to create the cosmetic appearance they desire?

Should the answer be "no" to any of these questions, then do not treat the patient. They may be insistent on you proceeding to treat them; however, this will not be in their best interests. Medical ethics dictates that such paternalism is undesirable in a successful relationship between a health care provider and a patient; however, in this situation, you are likely to confer harm to your patients and are unlikely to provide them any benefit. There is no shame in admitting that you do not have the necessary skills or equipment to successfully create the desired cosmetic outcome, and it is far better for all concerned for you to undertake the necessary further training before performing a treatment than simply *giving it a go.*

The appropriate communication skills, techniques, and contraindications to treatment are discussed later in this book. Please take the time to familiarise yourself with these to aid your development as a cosmetic practitioner.

## COMMON SKIN LESIONS AND HOW TO DESCRIBE THEM

Dermatology is a niche subject that many of us receive little formal training in, despite skin diseases being one of the most common complaints patients seek medical advice for. Before discussing common skin conditions, it is important to understand *how* to describe a skin lesion so you can accurately and concisely document findings in your notes as well as being able to liaise with a dermatologist should the situation necessitate it. You should always photograph skin lesions (with patient consent) to add to the medical record of your patients; being able to accurately describe them will aid anybody else who subsequently attends to them. Although a picture is worth a thousand words, a few choice words complement a picture tremendously.

Tables 6.1 through 6.6 outline common cutaneous lesions and how to appropriately describe them. It is worth noting that these findings are frequently not isolated; for example, you may encounter a maculopapular rash in a patient with measles.

## TABLE 6.1
## Flat Skin Lesions

| Description | Appearance | Diagram |
|---|---|---|
| Macule | Flat, non-palpable skin lesion <0.5–1 cm in diameter | |
| Patch | Flat, non-palpable skin lesion >1 cm in diameter | |

## TABLE 6.2
## Fluid-Filled Skin Lesions

| Description | Appearance | Diagram |
|---|---|---|
| Vesicle | 0.5–1-cm diameter blister containing clear fluid | |
| Bulla | Blister >1 cm in diameter containing clear fluid | |
| Pustule | Visible collection of pus <1 cm in diameter | |
| Abscess | Visible collection of pus >1 cm in diameter | |

## TABLE 6.3
## Raised Skin Lesions

| Description | Appearance | Diagram |
|---|---|---|
| Papule | Solid, raised lesion <0.5–1 cm in diameter | |
| Nodule | Solid, dome-shaped, raised lesion >1 cm in diameter | |
| Plaque | Large, superficial, flat-topped, palpable lesion | |
| Wheal | Blanching area of oedema within the dermis, usually >2 cm in diameter. Commonly associated with allergy and may have an erythematous border | |

**TABLE 6.4**
**Lesions with Skin Loss**

| Description | Appearance | Diagram |
|---|---|---|
| Atrophy | Epidermal/dermal thinning | |
| Fissure | Linear "crack" in the epidermis | |
| Erosion | Partial epidermal loss | |
| Ulcer | Complete epidermal with or without dermal loss | |

**TABLE 6.5**
**Characteristics of the Surface of Lesions**

| Description | Appearance | Diagram |
|---|---|---|
| Scale | White flakes on the surface of the lesion | |
| Excoriation | Scratch marks | |
| Lichenification | Epidermal thickening due to chronic scratching | |
| Crusting | Dried blood/pus/interstitial fluid | |

These tables should give you an arsenal of useful descriptive terms to help document and communicate your findings upon assessing your patient. For further understanding of associated skin conditions and how to describe them, it is advisable to consult a dedicated dermatology textbook.

## TABLE 6.6
## Vascular Changes within the Skin

| Description | Appearance | Diagram |
|---|---|---|
| Telangiectasia | Small, superficial, blanching blood vessels | |
| Petechiae | Tiny, non-blanching red/pink patches, usually pinhead-sized | |
| Purpura | Non-blanching red/pink patches which are larger than petechiae | |
| Spider naevus | Frond-like expansion of surface blood vessels | |
| Erythema | Blanching, red patch of skin | |
| Ecchymosis | Bruising | |

# COMMON BENIGN SKIN DISEASES

Skin diseases are very common, with more than 6 in every 10 people in the United Kingdom experiencing some form of skin disease at some point in their lives, with one in five appointments with general practitioners involving a complaint regarding the skin. Due to their prevalence, you will undoubtedly treat patients who have an active skin disease or have had them in the past. It is therefore imperative that you have an understanding of some of the more common skin complaints, their natural history and treatment regimes to allow you to both treat your cosmetic patients effectively and in a safe manner.

## ATOPIC ECZEMA

Atopic eczema is the most prevalent *endogenous* form of eczema and, as its name suggests, is often seen in conjunction with other atopic conditions such as hay fever and asthma. Approximately one in every five children in the United Kingdom develop atopic eczema at some point, and of those, six in every 10 will have symptoms which persist into adulthood. Although many people do grow out of this condition, it is worth noting that for the remainder it is a chronic disease which can be treated but not cured.

Historically the pathophysiology of atopic eczema was surprisingly poorly understood for such a common condition. It is now hypothesised to be a multisystem disorder, with genetic, immunological, barrier and environmental factors all contributing to its development. One very neat example of how these factors are all interlinked is that of the *FLG* gene, which codes for the epidermal protein filaggrin.

Filaggrin is a fascinating protein, which not only helps in regulating homeostasis and terminal differentiation of corneocytes but also aids in barrier formation, helps retain water within the epidermis and helps maintain a normal skin pH. Should filaggrin not function correctly, then the normal protective epidermal barrier can become inflamed and break down due to either a direct failure of the barrier itself or through the effects of pH imbalance or dehydration. The resultant inflammation it itchy, and this almost inevitably results in further barrier degradation due to patients inadvertently scratching afflicted areas. Breaks in the skin barrier expose the more delicate deep epidermis and dermis to irritants and opportunistic microbes, further potentiating the inflammatory response. It is hypothesised that allergens which manage to penetrate the damaged skin barrier can trigger an immunoglobulin E (IgE)–mediated allergic response, not only potentiating the localised inflammation but also propelling the development of other atopic sequelae such as asthma and hay fever.

The immune system also plays an important part in the development of atopic eczema, especially through the function of T-helper (TH) 2 lymphocytes. In cases of atopy, these lymphocytes secrete higher than normal levels of interleukin (IL)-4 and IL-5. IL-4 is important in the differentiation of naïve TH0 into TH2 lymphocytes, and therefore, an erroneously high circulating level of these cytokines results in an increased proportion of TH0 cells becoming TH2 lymphocytes. The functions of IL-5 are primarily concerned with B-lymphocyte growth, the production and secretion of IgA within mucous membranes and eosinophil activity. The clinical significance of the above is that a greater number of TH2 cells expressing these interleukins results in a greater, systemic inflammatory response as seen in other atopic conditions.

Clinically, atopic eczema presents with symmetrical, pruritic, ill-defined, erythematous patches with or without excoriations and weeping of serous fluid. Eczema is most commonly seen in flexural areas such as the antecubital fossae and backs of the knees; however, it is still commonly seen in the face and neck. In chronic cases, lichenification (thickening of the skin with increased skin markings) of the affected area may be seen due to repeated episodes of scratching. Other stigmata of chronic atopic eczema include hyperkeratosis and hyperpigmentation of the affected area.

Atopic eczema is routinely treated with thick emollients and topical steroids, with more potent steroids (such as betamethasone 0.1%) being used in flexural areas and less strong corticosteroids (such as 1% hydrocortisone) being reserved for more sensitive areas such as the face and hands.

As the skin barrier is disrupted in eczema, superadded infections are common, frequently caused by skin commensals such as *Staphylococcus aureus*. These infections are usually diagnosed clinically and can be tricky at times to distinguish from a simple flare in a patient's normal atopic eczema as the signs and symptoms will be very similar. In localised and uncomplicated cases of bacterial infection, a topical antibiotic such as fusidic acid may be used. Should the presentation be more severe, or should the patient fail to respond, then a two-week course of oral antibiotics, such as erythromycin or flucloxacillin, are frequently used in conjunction with topical treatments. Severe cases usually require hospital admission for specialist management.

Always bear in mind that infective exacerbations of eczema are not solely limited to bacteria and may also be caused by viruses such as *herpes simplex or molloscum contagiosum*, and fungi such as *Candida albicans*. Infected areas of eczema, especially by *Streptococcus* spp. can act as a superantigen, promoting the inflammatory response within and growth of pre-existing lesions as well as potentially the development of new foci of eczema elsewhere.

Regarding cosmetics, it is unsafe to treat a patient in close proximity to any eczematous areas, especially if they have an active flare or have recently had a deterioration in their symptoms. Treating an actively eczematous area will not only likely be highly irritating to your patient's skin but also confers a significantly elevated infection risk. Poor results may also be seen in patients who have chronically used topical steroids in the desired treatment area due to epithelial hypoplasia. These areas are best to be avoided, especially with dermal fillers, as there is an increased risk of an unsatisfactory cosmetic outcome due to a thinner overlying epidermal layer.

## Contact dermatitis

As its name suggests, contact dermatitis is an inflammatory response within the skin secondary to the direct contact of either an allergen or irritant substance. The nature of the trigger allows for further subdivision into either *irritant* or *allergic* contact dermatitis. A breakdown in the epidermal barrier commonly facilitates the development of this condition, and therefore, atopic eczema may predispose an individual to contact dermatitis. Other potential causes for impairment of the epidermal barrier and consequent contact dermatitis include extremes of age and direct trauma to the skin, such as in manual labourers.

## Irritant contact dermatitis

The crux of irritant contact dermatitis is epidermal trauma, frequently caused by the irritant itself. This condition rarely occurs with a single exposure and is far more likely should a person have repeated, sustained exposure to an irritant chemical. Repeated exposures often result in the natural oils on the skin surface being broken down and loss of moisture within the outer epidermal layers. A combination of these two effects results in skin being raw and cracked, allowing the irritants to penetrate deeper within the skin itself.

Irritant contact dermatitis frequently presents as a pruritic, erythematous patch. In severe cases, it may form fissures, blisters and bullae. Irritant contact dermatitis is frequently seen in the hands of an individual due to the likelihood of them using their hands to mix or administer irritant substances. Other common places to see this condition are the face, neck and arms; therefore, you are likely to encounter it at some point during your cosmetic practice.

There are multiple factors which can affect the severity of irritant contact dermatitis, with more severe cases typically being seen in the following situations:

- The *volume* of irritant is greater
- The *concentration* of irritant is greater
- *Increased length of time* exposed to the irritant
- *Increased frequency* of exposure to the irritant
- *Decreased* skin integrity
- Extremes of *temperature*
- Extremes of *humidity*

Irritant contact dermatitis is commonly associated with an individual's profession, especially those who work with caustic chemicals on a daily basis, such as hairdressers, nurses, surgeons and cleaners. Common causative agents include soaps, bleaches, detergents, cosmetics and polishes. It is worth bearing in mind that not all irritants are synthetic. Saliva is alkaline and repeated, prolonged exposures on the perioral skin can result in an individual developing "lip-lick eczema", which itself is a form of irritant contact dermatitis.

The core of managing irritant contact dermatitis is to avoid the irritant as best as possible. For some individuals, this is not possible due to the nature of their work, and subsequently, the next best approach is to limit exposure as much as possible through the use of personal protective equipment. Should a patient be symptomatic with pruritus and tenderness, then topical corticosteroids are frequently used in conjunction with a thick emollient to both act as a barrier and moisturise the traumatised skin. Finally, irritant contact dermatitis confers similar risks to superadded infection as atopic eczema and therefore it is a pertinent differential diagnosis in a person who continues to be symptomatic despite appropriate preventative and conservative management.

Any form of cosmetic treatment is contraindicated in a region of active irritant contact dermatitis, such as the treatment of hyperhidrosis in the hands with botulinum toxin or lip augmentation in a person with irritant contact dermatitis of the face. Treatment is contraindicated primarily due to the significantly elevated infection risk, as well as the possibility of prolonging a flare of irritant contact dermatitis due to further epidermal trauma. Counsel your patients about this and suggest they return for a further assessment once their skin has fully healed and they are no longer requiring any medication.

### ALLERGIC CONTACT DERMATITIS

Although similar in presentation to irritant contact dermatitis, the pathophysiology of allergic contact dermatitis is somewhat different. Rather than being triggered directly by an irritant on the skin, this form of dermatitis is a Type IV cell-mediated hypersensitivity reaction (see Chapter 13 for further information on the Coombs classification) with memory T cells previously exposed to the allergen secreting cytokines on subsequent exposures, triggering a characteristic erythematous, pruritic reaction. Allergic contact dermatitis, as with irritant contact dermatitis, is more likely to occur when there are breaks in the skin to allow causative allergens to penetrate deeper within the epidermis, and allergens deeper within the epidermis are more likely to be captured by antigen-presenting Langerhans cells. These cells are most prevalent within the stratum spinosum, and their capture and processing of allergens are one of the first steps in the hypersensitivity response.

In an acute outbreak of allergic contact dermatitis, the presentation is normally one of erythematous macules and papules if mild; however, in progressively more severe cases one may also see vesicles, blisters and bullae. Should a patient develop chronic form of this condition then commonly the affected skin will appear lichenified due to repeated rubbing with scaling, erythema and potentially a maculopapular rash.

Common allergens which trigger allergic contact dermatitis include nickel, chrome, perfume derivatives and drugs, such as neomycin and local anaesthetics. Unsurprisingly, the area in which a person usually first develops this condition are the areas which receive direct contact, such as the umbilical region if they were wearing a belt which contained nickel. It is possible, however, for areas distant from the site of contact to become affected through *autosensitisation*. The aetiology of this is not well understood and is hypothesised to be due to an immune response to the affected skin itself or due to circulating cytokines. Should a person become autosensitised, then they may present with an acute, symmetrical, generalised eczematous reaction with the arms, legs and trunk being most commonly involved. Presumably due to the systemic inflammatory response involved, a person who has an acute flare of autosensitisation often exhibits generalised malaise and fatigue with a low-grade fever.

The management of allergic contact dermatitis can be difficult simply because it can be hard to ascertain what the causative allergen is. Patients with suspected allergic contact dermatitis with no obvious trigger are commonly referred for patch testing to investigate this further. Once a causative allergen has been identified then the first line of management is to avoid it if at all possible. Acute flares are managed similarly to any other allergic response, with oral antihistamines such as chlorphenamine and topical steroids such as hydrocortisone comprising the mainstay of treatment. Allergic contact dermatitis respects the first rule of dermatology: "If it is dry, make it wet. If it is wet, make it dry" in that acute, weeping responses may benefit from the administration of topical agents to dry them out such as an aluminium acetate astringent, whereas dry, lichenified allergic contact dermatitis is usually best managed with a topical emollient.

## PSORIASIS

Psoriasis is a chronic, multisystem inflammatory condition with a typical skin presentation of well-defined, itchy, scaly, erythematous plaques with a white scale of dead erythrocytes. It is a relatively common condition, affecting up to one in 50 people. Although there are multiple different cutaneous presentations of psoriasis, the commonest form is *plaque psoriasis*, which affects up to nine in every 10 people with this condition. Psoriatic plaques frequently form on the scalp, elbows, knees, lower back and buttocks.

The clinical appearances of psoriasis are elegantly explained by the underlying pathogenesis. Psoriasis is mediated by both T-helper and T-cytotoxic lymphocytes which become activated by an unknown gene product or antigen. One hypothesised cause is erroneous autoactivation of T cells by an antimicrobial peptide called LL-37/cathelicidin, which is produced by keratinocytes and inflammatory cells in response to bacterial infection or trauma. These autoactivated T cells secrete pro-inflammatory cytokines, such as IL-17 and TNF-γ, which trigger hyperplasia, or an increased rate of cellular reproduction, in areas affected by psoriasis. The increased rate of epidermal cell turnover is quite striking, with keratinocytes in psoriatic plaques, taking only 4 days from maturation to shedding, whereas in normal skin it is closer to 28 days. These rapidly dividing cells end up stacking on top of one another, creating the characteristic raised plaques seen in psoriasis. It is a layer of dead keratinocytes which have not yet been shed that form the grey scale seen atop the plaques.

The erythematous base of psoriatic plaques is easily explained by the pro-inflammatory nature of the condition. Affected keratinocytes secrete vascular endothelial growth factor (VEGF) which drives angiogenesis to upregulate blood flow to affected areas. It is these new vessels which give the characteristic erythematous appearance underlying psoriatic plaques.

The chronicity of psoriasis is explained by a process known as a *positive chemotactic feedback loop*; where pro-inflammatory chemokines such as the aforementioned IL-17 and TNF stimulates keratinocytes to synthesise a further chemotactic agent known as *chemokine C-C motif ligand 20* (CCL20). CCL20 attracts T-lymphocytes to a psoriatic plaque, and on arrival, they are stimulated themselves to secrete more pro-inflammatory chemokines. The overall effect of this is one of perpetual inflammation, with a constant supply of T-lymphocytes which are autoactivated to secrete inflammatory chemokines and maintain a permanent inflammatory state.

As previously mentioned, psoriasis is not simply a cutaneous disease, with other inflammatory condition, such as psoriatic arthropathy and Crohn's disease being frequently associated. Psoriatic arthropathy is by far the most likely associated condition, affecting approximately one in every 10 people with psoriasis. This is frequently an asymmetrical, distal polyarthropathy of the small joints of the hands; however, it may also be present in the spine, sacroiliac joints and larger joints of the appendicular skeleton. The consequences of a persistent pro-inflammatory state also put those with psoriasis at a heightened risk of developing the metabolic syndrome, cardiovascular disease and type II diabetes mellitus. It is also worth appreciating that psoriasis not only confers a significant risk to a person's physical health but also their mental health. Any chronic condition causes an increased risk of mental illnesses such as depression to an individual, and psoriasis is no different. Some research suggests that those who have depression triggered by psoriasis may exhibit an improvement in their mood simply by treating psoriasis itself.

Psoriasis is a chronic condition which cannot be cured; therefore, the mainstay of treatment of its cutaneous manifestations is usually in controlling, as opposed to curing it. Limited psoriasis is commonly treated with topical agents, the first line of which is usually a thick emollient. Emollients are useful for symptomatic relief, as well as decreasing the visibility of the characteristic scales. It is worth noting that as they soften the outer epidermis, moisturisers allow for better absorption of other topical agents. Alongside emollients, other treatments often used include topical Vitamin D3 analogues, such as calcitriol, coal tar lotion and topical corticosteroids. One particular drawback of topical corticosteroids for psoriasis is that many patients suffer rebound psoriasis should they stop using them suddenly. Aside from medical management, sunlight (or ultraviolet [UV] light therapy) often confer symptomatic benefits to psoriasis patients. This is not to say that they should be advised to seek direct sunlight without appropriate skin protection; however, many of your patients may report the visibility and itchiness of plaques improves in the summer months. They should still be advised to be safe when they in the sun as they not only have the same risk of cancer and photoaging due to UV light as the normal population but the overstimulation with UV light may also trigger a flare of psoriasis symptoms. Finally, it is worth bearing in mind that patients with severe psoriasis or other associated autoimmune conditions, such as psoriatic arthritis or inflammatory bowel disease, may be taking systemic immunosuppressive medications, thus conferring a heightened infection risk with any invasive treatments.

One key consideration in the context of cosmetic treatments with those with psoriasis is that of the *Köbner phenomenon*, the formation of new foci of psoriasis in areas which have sustained cutaneous trauma. You must therefore inform patients with psoriasis that by traumatising the skin, such as with botulinum toxin or dermal filler administration, that you may, in fact, cause them to develop psoriasis at your treatment areas. The chances of this occurring are greater if your patients have previously developed new plaques at the site of cuts and abrasions in the past, and it is advisable to avoid treating anyone with a history of Köbnerisation.

## ACNE VULGARIS

Often associated with teenage skin, acne vulgaris is a disfiguring skin condition which arises from the *pilosebaceous unit*; a structure comprised of a hair, its follicle, arrector pili muscle and a sebaceous gland. It is so tremendously common it may almost be perceived as a normal part of adolescence, affecting almost 9 in every 10 teenagers, half of whom continue to have skin lesions which persist long into adulthood.

Although acne may be commonly misconstrued as simply lots of spots, it is, in fact, a complex condition comprising abnormal keratinisation, altered hormone levels, bacterial growth and a hypersensitive immune response. During puberty, androgen levels increase rapidly with resultant increased epidermal cell turnover and production of sebum by sebaceous glands. A combination of these two events result in the formation of *microcomedones*, plugs which block the pilosebaceous unit. Under normal circumstances, defunct keratinocytes are shed from the skin surface; however, as sebum is sticky, it causes them to aggregate and block the pilosebaceous unit from which they arise, creating the aforementioned microcomedones (Figure 6.1).

Despite being blocked, sebaceous glands continue to produce sebum, despite it having no clear route of drainage. This may be an occult process, with the pilosebaceous unit slowly increasing in size within the dermis, unbeknownst to the patient. This process is further compounded by the effects of bacteria, such as *Propionibacterium acnes*, which feed off the oily sebum and as a by-product of

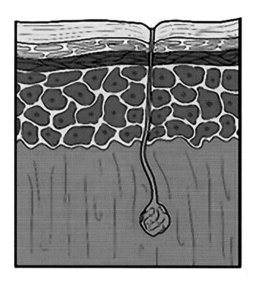

FIGURE 6.1    The pilosebaceous complex.

this produces the pro-inflammatory protein complex NF-KB and the production of leukotrienes through the activation of the enzyme 5-lipoxygenase. The inflammatory response to *P. acnes* results in the formation of pustules as immune cells are drawn to the infected pilosebaceous units to try and destroy the bacterial infection. These pustules appear as small white pockets of fluid which commonly have a surrounding erythematous reaction, forming the characteristic lesions seen in acne. Should the pressure within an infected pilosebaceous gland become too great, then these lesions may spontaneously erupt with the infection draining spontaneously. Sadly, for the patient, the localised pockets of inflammation caused by *P. acnes* can be quite severe when infections track deeper into the dermis. These deeper infections are not only more difficult to treat but are also likely to result in permanent scarring.

The diagnosis of acne vulgaris is usually clinical, with a physician identifying the presence of comedones. Comedones are something with which almost every one of us is *au fait*; however, they are more commonly referred to as "whiteheads" or "blackheads" when describing their macroscopic appearance. The underlying physiology of these two distinct types of comedone is essentially the same, with a microcomedone obstructing the pilosebaceous unit. The key differentiator as to which type of comedone will form is dependent on the level at which a microcomedone obstructs the unit. Should a microcomedone form deep within the pilosebaceous unit, then oxygen will not be able to reach the underlying mixture of dead keratinocytes and sebum and they will remain white, thus forming a "whitehead". Should the microcomedone be causing a more distal obstruction, however, then oxygen will reach the dead keratinocytes and oxidise melanin within them. This reaction causes the melanin to turn black and unsurprisingly forming "blackheads".

Sadly, acne treatments may take up to four months from initiation to have an appreciable benefit. The treatment regimens offered to patients with acne are dictated by disease severity. In mild acne, patients are often offered an astringent such as topical benzoyl peroxide lotion as well as topical antibiotics such as erythromycin or clindamycin. Should these topical treatments prove ineffective, or if a person has moderate acne on presentation, then a 16-week course of oral antibiotics such as lymecycline or oxytetracycline are often advised in conjunction with benzoyl peroxide. Female patients may also have some benefit from taking the combined oral contraceptive pill to decrease circulating testosterone levels and subsequently decreasing sebum production. Severe cases should be managed by a consultant dermatologist for consideration of isotretinoin, a vitamin A analogue, which induces apoptosis within sebaceous glands. It is usually a very effective medication with over 8 in every 10 patients reporting resolution of acne lesions after a 20-week treatment regime. Isotretinoin should only be dispensed by a consultant dermatologist as it has a considerable side-effect profile, including mucosal dryness, worsening of acne, depression and psychosis. It is also a potent teratogenic agent, and females of childbearing age should *always* have adequate contraception whilst on this treatment.

Anecdotal evidence suggests that botulinum toxin may help decrease the prominence of comedones and pustules seen in acne. This is due to chemical denervation of muscarinic receptors within sebaceous glands due to chemical denervation of acetylcholine secreting neurones. In turn, there is resultant decreased sebum production in the skin surrounding the injection sites for up to 16 weeks. Decreased sebum production often correlates with decreased pustulosis and comedone formation, the hallmarks of acne vulgaris. Conversely, dermal filler treatments are inadvisable in areas which have acne pustules in close proximity, due to conferring a heightened infection risk and an increased likelihood of pushing bacteria such as *P. acnes* deeper within the soft tissues of the face.

## CUTANEOUS MALIGNANCIES

Skin cancers such as malignant melanoma are the fifth-most common malignancy in the United Kingdom, and with more people using sunbeds and travelling abroad to sunny locales, the incidence of skin cancer is expected to increase in the near future. As with almost all cancers, early detection and treatment correlate with increased survival rates. As a cosmetic practitioner, you may be the only person who undertakes a dedicated dermatological assessment on a patient, and it is vital to be able to identify some of the more common skin cancers to allow your patients to have swift and appropriate management. If you are unsure of whether a patient has a cutaneous malignancy, it is strongly advisable to err on the side of caution and advise them to see their general practitioner for further assessment. As a cosmetic practitioner you are not expected to manage these patients, but it is wholly unethical to do nothing about any you may encounter. The gold standard for diagnosis of any malignancy is to have a tissue diagnosis from histopathological investigations. It is for this reason that it is strongly unadvisable to ever perform the removal of any moles or skin blemishes in a cosmetic practice unless you are appropriately trained to do so, are certain you will achieve clear margins and can arrange for the appropriate histopathological, radiological and medical follow-up.

In this chapter, we outline some of the more common premalignant and malignant cutaneous tumours to be aware of when assessing your patients.

## PREMALIGNANT TUMOURS: SOLAR KERATOSIS

Solar keratoses are premalignant tumours arising from the stratum basale and occur almost exclusively in sun-damaged skin and appear as brownish-red patches on areas which have been exposed to the sun (such as the face or helix of the ear). The patient may describe these as itchy, although commonly they are asymptomatic. Some solar keratoses are raised and may have a "warty appearance" due to epidermal hypertrophy and are subsequently known as *hypertrophic solar keratoses*. Should a solar keratosis become indurated, inflamed or ulcerated, then this may be an indication that they are transforming into a malignant squamous cell carcinoma. Such transformations are rare, occurring in fewer than one in 1,000 solar keratoses; however, this should still not be overlooked. Most solar keratoses are not problematic for patients and require no specific treatment, with one in five spontaneously regressing. Advise any patients with solar keratoses to monitor their skin as their presence indicates chronic UV damage with a subsequence increased risk of skin cancer formation.

## PREMALIGNANT TUMOURS: BOWEN'S DISEASE

Unlike solar keratoses, Bowen's disease is a premalignant tumour which arises from dysplastic changes throughout the entire epidermis. It is likely that as they have a greater number of epidermal layers involved, they are more susceptible to becoming malignant, with up to 5% of these premalignant tumours undergoing malignant transformation into squamous cell carcinomas. As is the case with solar keratoses, one of the key determinants in the development of Bowen's disease is excessive sun exposure with them frequently presenting on sun-exposed areas.

The characteristic appearances of Bowen's disease are a well-defined erythematous scaly or warty plaque with a flat edge and, like solar keratoses, any nodularity or ulceration is suggestive of transformation into a squamous cell carcinoma. As these lesions have a relatively high rate of becoming malignant, it is strongly advisable that you refer them to their general practitioner to arrange for further assessment, which likely will include a skin biopsy.

## MALIGNANT TUMOURS: SQUAMOUS CELL CARCINOMA

Squamous cell carcinomas (SCCs) of the skin are the second-most common skin cancer, comprising approximately one in five skin cancers (not including melanoma). They commonly appear as a keratotic or ulcerated nodule with a rolled border and a granulomatous base and have increased incidence in the elderly and in males. Their prognosis is linked to the chance of metastasis, which is related to the anatomical location of the tumour as well as the host immune status, with immunocompromised patients being both more likely to develop a SCC as well as having lesions which metastasise to other sites. It may be surprising to some that the risk of metastasis of SCC is lower in sun-exposed areas, with a greater metastatic potential in areas which are usually covered such as the sole of the foot. This does not mean you should disregard a potential SCC in a sun-exposed area, as they will require excision, histological grading and radiological staging to allow for appropriate further management.

## MALIGNANT TUMOURS: BASAL CELL CARCINOMAS

These tumours are the commonest skin cancers. They are slow-growing and locally invasive, yet metastases are almost unheard of. The most common demographic to develop a basal cell carcinoma (BCC) is middle-aged Caucasians. There are four main types of BCC, as outlined in Table 6.7.

---

**TABLE 6.7**
**Basal Cell Carcinoma (BCC) Subtypes**

| Description | Appearances |
| --- | --- |
| Nodulocystic | Most commonly found on the face or neck, these dome-shaped papules with a "pearly" appearance and associated telangiectasia. If left untreated for a long time, they may become ulcerated with rolled edges. These are colloquially known as "rodent ulcers". |
| Superficial | These BCCs are most commonly seen on the trunk and present as scaly erythematous plaques. |
| Pigmented | These BCCs contain flecks of melanin, and if heavily pigmented, they may mimic a malignant melanoma. Inspect these lesions closely for a pearly appearance which may help you differentiate these two malignancies. |
| Morphoeic | These BCCs are waxy, indurated plaques which may resemble a scar. |

---

As with an SCC, the gold standard management of a BCC is excision with histological analysis.

## MALIGNANT TUMOURS: MALIGNANT MELANOMA

Malignant melanoma frequently arises in patients younger than age 50, are more common in males and are the commonest cancer in young adults. Despite being the least common cutaneous malignancy, malignant melanoma confers by have the worst prognosis, causing almost three-quarters of all deaths from skin cancer.

Being melanomatous in origin, malignant melanomas are pigmented lesions, and you should suspect it in *any funny-looking mole*. A simple tool to use in assessing a potential malignant melanoma is the ABCDEF criteria:

**A**symmetrical outline
**B**order irregularity
**C**olour variation within the lesion with shades of black, brown or pink
**D**iameter over 6 mm

**E**volution, with the mole changing in size, shape, or colour
**F**unny-looking mole – does it simply look *odd*?

Seeing any of the preceding should raise your suspicion for a potential malignant melanoma and would warrant further assessment by a specialist.

As with BCCs, there are also several subtypes of malignant melanoma, including those described in Table 6.8.

---

**TABLE 6.8**
**Common Subtypes of Malignant Melanoma**

| Description | Appearances |
|---|---|
| Superficial spreading melanoma | The commonest subtype, presenting as an irregular, slowly enlarging, slightly raised, pigmented plaque. Nodularity may signify a deeper invasion. |
| Nodular melanoma | These melanomas are unsurprisingly nodular in appearance and grow rapidly and invade deeply. They may be amelanotic, lacking (but not completely devoid of) pigment. |
| Lentigo maligna melanoma | These melanomas arise from a slow-growing melanoma in situ called a lentigo maligna and are commonly associated with chronic ultraviolet light damage. These melanomas are the most frequently encountered on the face and frequently appear as a nodular lesion with a spreading superficial border. |

---

As with all other skin cancers, malignant melanomas require urgent specialist assessment. Should you spot a funny-looking mole, it is always worth advising your patent to see their general practitioner urgently to arrange for the necessary investigations and treatment. Your patient may have *only one chance* to have their cancer promptly diagnosed and treated to decrease the chance of fatal metastatic disease.

## BODY DYSMORPHIA

Body dysmorphia is a psychiatric condition characterised by a person's inability to appreciate their true physical appearance, and they will often spend a significant portion of their time critiquing their looks, picking up on subtleties that are often unnoticeable to others. Some of the flaws that a person claims to have may not be present whatsoever, which would be in keeping with a delusional state.

Body dysmorphia affects both men and women and is of a greater prevalence in teenagers and young adults, affecting approximately 25 people in every 1,000. It is likely to be significantly underdiagnosed like many other mental health disorders and therefore those who suffer with it may be unaware of this diagnosis and presume that their response to their physical appearance is a normal reaction.

A person with body dysmorphia may have one or more of the following signs:

• Spending a lot of time worrying about their appearance
• Spending a lot of time worrying about how others perceive their appearance

- Obsessing over their appearance in mirrors (or even avoiding mirrors altogether)
- Spending a lot of time trying to conceal their perceived flaws

The preceding signs are obviously quite weak to create a definite diagnosis, as they can all be perceived as a natural thing to do. It is unlikely to ever meet a person who hasn't, at some point or another, compared themselves to another individual or been worried about being seen as attractive. The primary difference between body dysmorphia and normal angst about one's appearance is that in body dysmorphia, what may be a normal level of concern for an individual becomes an obsession which takes up significant amounts of their time and consumes their thoughts.

In the realms of cosmetic medicine, every person who presents to you will be doing so because there is an aspect of themselves they do not like and wish to change. You need to screen every patient you see carefully to ascertain just how much the thing they wish to alter is affecting their life. In true body dysmorphia, patients will be consumed by these flaws, may spend several hours every day obsessing over them and may report intrusive, negative thoughts. Body dysmorphia is not simply vanity. It is a mental disorder which requires specialist treatment. When you are consenting a person for a procedure, take the time to explore the number of procedures they have had beforehand and how effective the person perceived them to be. In body dysmorphia, patients may seek cosmetic treatments of multiple types from many different practitioners but will rarely be satisfied with the results as the underlying obsessions have not been treated. Ask a person about the aforementioned four major signs and ask how much time each day is spent thinking about their appearance and focusing on perceived physical flaws. Should they inform you that they spend a significant amount of their time obsessing over their appearance or how others view them then it is not advisable to continue with treatment. If you are not a fully qualified psychiatrist with the necessary skills to treat and follow-up this condition, politely decline to treat them and advise they see their general practitioner to get it addressed. Successful identification and treatment of body dysmorphic disorder can be a life-saving intervention, as it confers a high rate of both suicidal ideation and suicide attempts.

# 7 Communication skills

Communication is hardwired into all of us. Human beings are inherently social creatures and effective communication is essential to maintain and develop the strong bonds we form with family and friends throughout our lives. Our first forays into communicating with others starts in the newborn period, with babies communicating to others through crying to get the food, attention and reassurance they require. As we age, our communication strategies become more refined, from smiling at and seeking eye contact with close family members at around two months of age to babbling simple words from nine months or so to pointing at desirable objects and people from one year old. These developmental milestones are not set in stone as every baby is different; however, most children progress in a similar pattern to this as their neurolinguistic skills develop. From the age of two, many children will be constructing simple sentences which become more complex as they become older. As children reach school age, a significant number can actively listen, follow instructions, recite information and hold a conversation with others. It is utterly fascinating to consider that within four short years, we go from having crying as our sole source of communication to actively verbalising our dreams and desires with others.

We are not solely limited to direct communication through verbal cues, however with body language, written text and pictorial methods of communication also playing an integral role in our lives. Children frequently draw pictures to demonstrate what interests them most, and as our ability to write progresses, pictures are frequently superseded with writing. Writing allows us to communicate our ideas with other people indefinitely, leaving a permanent reminder of how we felt at a particular time. Written text is a fantastic method of communication as it allows us to potentially share our thoughts and feelings with people all over the world through letters, emails and social media.

As we age our communication skills continue to develop, adhering to cultural and societal norms as well as learning how to approach more difficult individuals. Learning how to resolve conflict from a young age sets us up for a lifetime of negotiating and diffusing awkward situations. Many of us, however, cannot put a finger on a specific time where we learned how to do all of this, and on reflection, if we think back to how we were as children and teenagers, our abilities to communicate undoubtedly change as we mature.

The ability to communicate effectively is at the core of all cosmetic practice, encompassing both verbal and non-verbal communication as well as with pictures and in writing. In almost any consultation you conduct, you will be the *expert opinion* on cosmesis. Being able to break down complex ideas in a simple and tactful manner may require diagrams to illustrate your point, as well as explaining a potentially complicated written consent form. If you are unable to help your patient to understand the treatments you are proposing (or indeed advising against), then your patients cannot give informed consent, which may result in disastrous consequences. In this chapter, we explore the importance of effective communication, as well as key communication skills to add to your repertoire to allow you to practise cosmetics both safely and ethically.

DOI: 10.1201/9781003198840-7

## THE IMPORTANCE OF BODY LANGUAGE

Body language makes up over 90% of all human communication and primarily consists of subconscious cues to express one person's feelings to others without a word being said. One brief experiment to prove just how sensitive we are to body language is to watch a television programme with the sound turned off. You may surprise yourself as to how easily you can interpret an actor's emotions without the need to hear what they are saying. As body language is primarily subconscious, many of us will unwittingly give away whether we enjoy the company or conversation of another through non-verbal cues. Learning how to manage your body language in the setting of a medical consultation is vital in building a good rapport with your patients, which, in turn, will create a stronger practitioner–patient relationship with better outcomes.

Research reminds us that patients closely observe their doctors for not only what is being said but also regarding their body language during a consultation. One observational study highlighted that the degree of eye contact was perceived by patients to correlate with the level of interest a doctor had in them, and a lack of eye contact was particularly bothersome to younger and more well-educated patients. Further research demonstrated that doctors who had a more engaging posture and maintained better eye contact were likely to have more information volunteered to them by patients than those who did the opposite. This implies that having an open, upright posture and maintaining eye contact are not only good manners but also good practices. The utilisation of body language and posture can not only allow for you to garner useful information from patients but also from those who demonstrate good eye contact, head nods and gestures, positive position and an engaging tone of voice have improved patient satisfaction and understanding, heightened awareness of emotional distress, and lower rates of litigation.

Some examples of positive and negative body language are listed in Table 7.1.

---

**TABLE 7.1**
**Examples of Positive and Negative Body Language**

| Positive Body Language | Negative Body Language |
| --- | --- |
| • Greeting patients in the waiting room | • Calling patients in from our office |
| • Shaking your patient's hand | • Not standing or shaking hands on arrival |
| • Maintaining eye contact | • Avoiding eye contact |
| • Having a neutral or slightly happy facial ex-pression (should the consultation dictate it). If your patient is visibly distressed, then smiling or neutrality is unlikely to be looked on favourably! | • Looking serious or stern |
| | • Not mirroring facial cues |
| | • Slouching or leaning back |
| • Sitting upright and slightly leaning towards the patient | • Crossed arms or legs |
| • Open posture | • Staring blankly whilst being spoken to |
| • Nodding whilst the patient is talking | • Touching your face is seen as being untrustworthy |
| • Gesturing with your hands whilst talking | |

One important factor to consider in a medical consultation is the distraction of patient notes, be that taking them whilst a patient is talking or reviewing them during a consultation. Patients may believe that you reading your notes is a sign of disinterest in them, and therefore, this is a facet of your consultation that you should manage accordingly. It is advisable to deliberately avoid looking at patient notes until you have listened to their opening statement and taken your initial history. Once this has happened, signpost to your patient that you need to briefly review or update their notes with what has been said. This will help your patient to understand your thought processes, as well as feeling that they have supplied you with valuable information. Try to keep note reading in front of the patient to a minimum and refresh yourself with their history *before* they have entered your consultation room. Once you have finished writing in their notes, inform them that you are listening once more and revert to the positive non-verbal cues previously outlined. If you spend ages fawning over notes or not interacting with patients without informing them why you are doing so, they will frequently believe you are either disinterested in them or that you do not value their time or presence in your practice.

Despite being a subconscious act, body language is nonetheless a skill which we can practice to incorporate into our interactions with others. We all have the innate ability to detect insincerity, such as a fake smile or crocodile tears. Your patients are not ignorant, and if you do not truly believe what you are saying or doing, then they will pick up on this to the detriment of your relationship. Practising medical consultations (including body language) with a friend will allow you to fine-tune these skills. Ensure they give you honest feedback so you can further develop your nonverbal communication.

## TAKING A FOCUSED MEDICAL HISTORY WITH THE CALGARY–CAMBRIDGE MODEL

Accurately taking and recording a medical history is a fundamental part of your cosmetic practice. Should you wish to have a practice of the highest esteem, then you will need to have succinct and factual notes for auditing purposes in the future. Having an accurate patient record is not only a legal requirement but also crucial for follow-up treatments and auditing purposes in the unfortunate event of a dissatisfied patient or should you make a mistake. If you are not accustomed to taking a medical history then it may feel a bit clunky or artificial at first; however, with time and practice, it will become second nature and roll off your tongue.

The Calgary–Cambridge model is taught in UK medical schools and is a fantastic tool to lean back on when you are starting out or should you forget what to ask next (Figure 7.1). Over time, you will undoubtedly modify this to what works best for you and your patients, which is absolutely fine.

### Initiating the session

Many people who come to you for treatments will be nervous, especially if it is their first foray into the world of cosmetic medicine. In my experience, the two most common fears when someone comes into my office is the fear of the unknown and

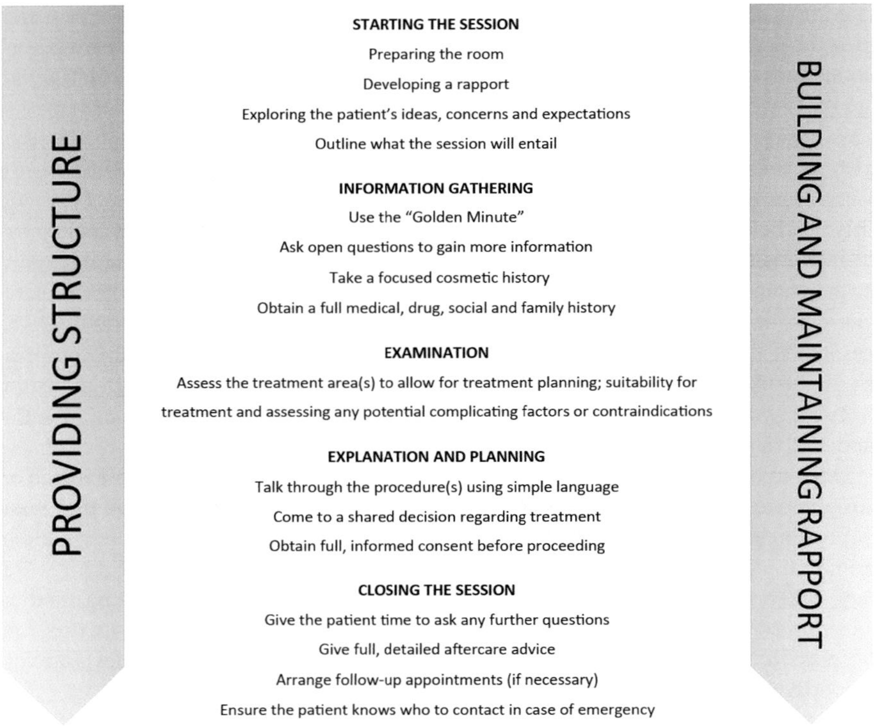

PROVIDING STRUCTURE

BUILDING AND MAINTAINING RAPPORT

**STARTING THE SESSION**

Preparing the room

Developing a rapport

Exploring the patient's ideas, concerns and expectations

Outline what the session will entail

**INFORMATION GATHERING**

Use the "Golden Minute"

Ask open questions to gain more information

Take a focused cosmetic history

Obtain a full medical, drug, social and family history

**EXAMINATION**

Assess the treatment area(s) to allow for treatment planning; suitability for
treatment and assessing any potential complicating factors or contraindications

**EXPLANATION AND PLANNING**

Talk through the procedure(s) using simple language

Come to a shared decision regarding treatment

Obtain full, informed consent before proceeding

**CLOSING THE SESSION**

Give the patient time to ask any further questions

Give full, detailed aftercare advice

Arrange follow-up appointments (if necessary)

Ensure the patient knows who to contact in case of emergency

**FIGURE 7.1**    Amended Calgary–Cambridge model for cosmetic practice.

the fact that needles are involved! Try to put them at ease when they attend. Spend time to talk to them about their journey, the weather, their job, pets, anything! A few minutes of small talk will work wonders in temporarily alleviating their initial fears and will allow them to settle down somewhat so you can start your consultation and help them offer and retain the relevant information to allow you to proceed.

Once your patient is settled, outline what you will be discussing today. Let them know you will be taking a medical history, which will remain confidential, and then outline which procedures you will discuss (based on what they have attended to have done). This way they won't be taken by surprise and will hopefully allow your consultation to flow nicely.

### INFORMATION GATHERING

First of all, ask your patient an open question, such as "What brings you in today?" Try to not interrupt for one minute. This technique is known as the *golden minute*, and it is a very useful tool to allow a person to share far more information than should you be interrupting every few seconds with your own input. Use non-verbal cues, such as nodding and smiling, to encourage them to keep talking. Obviously if you are with a patient who is not overly loquacious, then this strategy does not work all too well. If your patient offers you two sentences and then stops talking, there is little benefit to sitting in silence with them until the minute is up.

Important questions to ask in the initial stages of the consultation are whether they have had previous treatments before, when, by whom and how well it worked. If a person has had multiple unsatisfactory outcomes by a range of practitioners, then have the idea of body dysmorphic disorder in the back of your mind, especially considering this condition is an absolute contraindication to cosmetic treatments. Should you not suspect body dysmorphia, then it is advisable to use your own judgement on when their last treatment was performed and by whom before deciding to proceed. A good rule to adhere to is to advise no further dermal filler augmentation within four months of the previous treatment and no botulinum toxin therapy within three months (unless there has been a complication which mandates further treatment). This is to not only allow an individual to get accustomed to their new appearance, but fewer injections will decrease the risk of complications such as infection, over-filling and scarring.

Once you have taken a brief cosmetic history, take the time to take a focused medical history. In particular ask about the following:

- Recent skin infections including cold sores
- Recent dental work or dental infection
- Recent oral/facial surgery
- Recent systemic illness
- Any immunosuppressive conditions such as diabetes mellitus or HIV
- Is there a chance they are pregnant/are they breastfeeding?

Once you are satisfied that your patient has no absolute contraindications to treatment, proceed to ask them about any medications they may be taking (see the section on immunomodulatory drugs for further information). Explore any allergies they may have, including to latex should you be using latex gloves. If you are ever unsure as to whether your product contains a particular allergen, then it is worthwhile contacting the manufacturer before you treat a patient to confirm or deny their presence.

The social history is quite important in advising your patients on how long a treatment will last. Smoking, drinking, extreme exercise and excessive ultraviolet light will result in your treatments not lasting as long. Inform your patients of this, so they will be well aware that should treatments only be apparent for a shorter time than anticipated, then it may be due to their lifestyle. Take the time to ask them about their dietary habits and exercise regimes too. Malnourishment results in poor-quality skin and increases the chances of infection. Ask your patient when they next intend to exercise, as it is inadvisable to exercise for the remainder of the day after treatment due to the risk of infection and a poor cosmetic effect due to vasodilation, especially regarding botulinum toxin treatment. You should take this opportunity to advise your patients on the benefit of a healthy lifestyle going forward to decrease both the medical and outward signs of ageing.

Finally take a brief family history. Much of this is irrelevant; if a patient's 101-year-old grandmother has osteoarthritis, it is unlikely to impact on the efficacy or safety of your treatment. A good way to ask about family history is *"Are you aware of any conditions which run in your family affecting people of your age?"* which is a broad stroke screening tool to highlight any pertinent conditions. Once you have done that, ask specifically about diabetes, neuromuscular and mental health disorders as these may be familial. Finally ask if anyone who lives with them has had any recent infectious diseases, as it may be that they are currently in the incubation period of an infection which would contravene your treatment.

## PHYSICAL EXAMINATION

You are not expected to auscultate a patient's chest or check their nails for clubbing, but you do need to examine the treatment area. Ask your patient for permission to have a close look and pop on some gloves. Carefully examine the area which they want treatment, assessing for signs of infection, spots or skin breaks. If they have had dermal fillers in that area before, check carefully for lumps, granulomas, scarring or anything else which will interfere with your cosmetic result or put the patient at undue risk of further complications. When assessing an area for dermal fillers, consider in your head whether the desired cosmetic outcome can be created and the best way to go about doing so. If you are convinced that you cannot give your patient the treatment or cosmetic outcome they are seeking, then a thorough examination will give you the information you need to explain to your patient that proceeding with treatment is not in their best interests.

In the context of botulinum toxin, assess for the level of movement and underlying muscle bulk, as well as check for a shiny appearance of the skin which may reflect overtreatment in the past. Check for dynamic and static lines, as static lines may have a reduced appearance after treatment but are unlikely to go altogether.

Once you have assessed the treatment area, assess the face as a whole so you can plan what you wish to do to treat a patient. Sometimes they will present wanting a particular outcome but have been misled as to the best possible treatment for them. A prime example would be in peri-oral lines, where sometimes filling the lip is a better treatment than augmenting the lines themselves. Take the time to review your patient's face as a whole and assess their features to determine whether they are strong or subtle and how your treatment will affect their overall appearance.

Finally, when examining your patient check for large blood vessels which may prove tricky during treatment, as you do not want to accidentally cause a vascular occlusion or inject your product directly into a blood vessel. Taking the time to do a quick lymph node examination is also good practice, as they may point to an underlying pathology not obvious at a cursory glance.

## EXPLANATION AND PLANNING

The world of cosmetics is completely nebulous to the majority of the public. Many people will turn up wanting to look a certain way without an appreciation of how this appearance can be created. Once you have taken a history and assessed your patient, take the time to explain what your thoughts are in *plain English*. If you wish to offer some technical information, such as the level of cross-linking in dermal fillers, then take the time to slowly and clearly explain how a particular product works and why you would advise it. The use of technical terms or medical jargon is not advisable as many patients won't understand what you are discussing and may be too embarrassed to ask you to explain yourself further. If your patient does not understand what you are talking about, then they cannot offer informed consent, which we discuss later in this chapter.

It is good practice when explaining a treatment plan to a patient to ask them to hold a hand-held mirror in front of their face. First, ask your patient to further explain in as much detail as possible what they are hoping to achieve by pointing to the parts of their face they want altered. Once they have done so, ask them to look at themselves whilst you point out exactly *how* you intend to treat them based on their request. demonstrate areas which you intend to treat and those you intend to leave alone with the patient focusing on themselves in the mirror. This will give them a far greater insight into your thought processes than will you trying to explain in technical terms what you intend to do and allow your patients to give true informed consent. After you have done this, double-check with the patient that you are both in agreement before proceeding and offer them ample time to discuss any further questions they may have.

### CLOSING THE SESSION

In this setting, you are not really closing the session *per se*, you are merely getting ready to begin your treatments. This may be, however, a patient's last opportunity to ask any questions before you begin your treatments. Ask your patient if there is anything else they would like to ask, or anything which is unclear. It is useful to make it a bit lighthearted so they do not feel impolite. State that you are aware that you often explain things poorly (even if you are an expert explainer!) and implore them to seek clarification on any points you have made. This will make them more likely to be open about anything they find unclear and will allow you to proceed with treatments knowing that your patient has had ample opportunity to understand and appreciate your treatment strategy, and more important, they will be able to give proper informed consent.

## SHARED DECISION-MAKING

Any and all treatment plans should be developed as a consensus between you and your patient. They will have their own preconceived ideas of which treatments they would like and which outcomes they hope to achieve. Many patients will have done extensive research into the treatments they are after and will be very knowledgeable about the subject; however, most will not share the expert knowledge that you will have obtained during your time in practice. You must empower your patients by enhancing their understanding of treatments to involve them in planning their treatment regimes. Educate your patients during your consultation in order to bring them on a level with yourself to ensure they can be active partners in the decision-making process. Some patients may wish for you to take a paternalistic stance as they see you as *the expert*, yet as beauty is such a subjective field, it is imperative you strive to make any treatment decisions as a shared consensus.

A useful place to start in this process is to ask your patient what their understanding is of the treatments or outcomes they are after so that you pitch the information you give them at the correct level. It is as inadvisable to patronise your patient by "dumbing-down" information as it is to presume that they have the same level of knowledge as you. Take the time to explore their ideas, concerns and expectations for the treatment so you have useful points from which to construct your discussion.

Once you have ascertained your patient's level of knowledge, elicit their preferences and ideal outcome from a treatment for an in-depth discussion. Take the time to explore each in turn, discussing the positives and negatives of each one (including potential risks). Encourage your patient to ask questions during the discussion of each treatment and take the time to answer their questions in detail. A key tool to ensure that you cover as many bases as possible is to ask them their ideas, concerns and expectations for each treatment discussed. This will allow you to develop a holistic approach to addressing their concerns. Once you have talked about each potential treatment, take the time to summarise what you have discussed into a few short and easily digested sentences.

Despite your aim to empower your patients, you do not wish for them to feel alone in this process. You are the expert opinion in cosmetic therapy and therefore you are well within your right to advise them whether you think a particular treatment will benefit them or not. If your patient declines the most advisable treatment in favour of a less effective one, ask them their rationale for this in a non-confrontational matter. There are multiple reasons why a patient may choose a lesser treatment, such as the cost, or it may be simply that you have not explained the potential treatment strategy in enough detail.

Once you and your patient have had a frank discussion about the different treatment options available, ask them which they find the most favourable and why. Ascertain their preferences and decide along with them whether it is indeed in their best interests. During this process, you need to take into account your patient as a whole, including their lifestyle, cultural beliefs and background.

Finally, you need to ascertain that you have not coerced your patient into a treatment outcome they are not after. Take the time to recap what you have discussed and take into account the questions they have asked you and ensure you have addressed them in sufficient detail. At times you may find that at this point you and your patient still disagree, which is not uncommon in the case of patients wanting excessive treatment which you suspect is either unsafe or will not confer a successful cosmetic outcome. Should this occur, give them an information leaflet, encourage them to talk things through with a trusted family member or friend, and ask them to revisit you in a few weeks' time. This allows them to carefully think through your discussion to ensure that you are both in agreement that the best possible outcome can be achieved.

If you and your patient are unable to decide on a suitable treatment plan, then it is best practice to not proceed. Cosmetic treatments are never a necessity, and you should never coerce your patient to have a treatment they do not want to have or which will be unlikely to give them the desired outcome. Conversely, should your patient be desperate for a treatment which you fundamentally believe will not benefit them in any way, then feel free to decline to treat them. Every cosmetic treatment confers a degree of risk of harm to your patient; therefore, administering an ineffective or ill-advised treatment may only offer negative consequences.

## THE CONSENT PROCESS AND THE MONTGOMERY RULING

Informed consent is both an ethical and legal obligation should you intend to perform any procedure on a patient. In 2015, the Montgomery Ruling in 2015 has superseded the Bolam test as the benchmark case in the United Kingdom for medical negligence regarding consent. The ruling applies to healthcare providers to ensure that they "take reasonable care to ensure that the patient is aware of any material risks involved in any treatment, and of any reasonable alternative or variant treatments". A material risk is one in which "a reasonable person in the patient's position would be likely to attach significance to the risk, or the doctor is or should reasonably be aware that the particular patient would be likely to attach significance to it".

In practice, there are a plethora of ethical and legal reasons why you must achieve informed consent before initiating any intervention to a patient. Should you touch your patient in any way without gaining their express consent, then you have committed battery in the eyes of UK law. Ethically, it is not right to examine a person or give them a treatment without them understanding exactly why it is advised as your patient may simply *not want you to.*

The first step in obtaining informed consent is to ascertain whether your patient has the capacity to make decisions for themselves. The capacity assessment comprises of four parts, and to have capacity, your patient must be able to do the following:

- Understand the information you are giving them
- Use and weigh up the information
- Retain the information
- Express a decision

If your patient cannot do all the preceding points, they are deemed to lack capacity and therefore cannot consent to treatment. It is worth noting that a capacity assessment is only valid at the time it is taken, as a person may lose or gain capacity afterwards. Common reversible factors which may temporarily affect capacity include alcohol or drug intoxication, infections and low blood sugar in people with diabetes. Should you suspect your patient is not capacious, then do not proceed to treatment, even if they have already given written consent. One caveat to capacity is the right to make poor decisions; just because somebody makes an unwise decision it does not mean they lack capacity; however, should a patient insist on an unwise treatment then it is still advisable not to treat them.

Once you have ascertained your patient has capacity, it is then your duty to offer them all the relevant information they require to make an informed decision. Explore their prior knowledge of the desired treatment and then add to their knowledge in plain language to ensure they are aware of the likely outcomes of that treatment, any viable alternatives and what will happen if you simply do nothing. So you can be content in the knowledge that they understand what you have discussed you may wish to ask them to repeat the salient points back to clarify anything they do not understand fully. Once you have done this, ask them if they have any questions or anything they wish to discuss in more detail. Encourage them to share their ideas, concerns and expectations about the treatment so you can address each in turn before beginning treatment.

Explaining risk comes in two distinct phases; the first is the likelihood of a risk occurring, and the second is the significance of said risk. When explaining the likelihood of a risk avoid using percentages and instead use absolute numbers as research suggests that this is easier for patients to comprehend and remember. Use relatable numbers, such as "1 in 100 people undergoing this procedure may expect to experience . . ." so your patients can visualise the chances of an adverse event happening to them. Never trivialise risk, as some people may see 1 in 100 as a relatively low risk, whereas others may see it as far too high. Severity of risk is just as important as the chance of a complication occurring. If we were to consider dermal filler treatment, the risk of blindness or embolus causing stroke are minute; however, the potential morbidity and mortality from these events are staggeringly high. This is why it is essential to inform patients of all serious risks so they can truly make an informed decision. Bear in mind that in respect to cosmesis, an undesirable outcome is arguably the most common risk you may incur. A poor cosmetic outcome is unlikely to kill or permanently disable your patient, but it may still have severe negative psychological consequences on them. *Always* consent your patient that an undesirable outcome may happen as you be unable to create your patient's desired look or may have misunderstood what they are after.

Written consent is essential before undertaking any cosmetic treatment. It is good practice to supply your patient with a consent form outlining the potential benefits and risks of the treatment so they can read it and recap your discussion before consenting to proceed. One way you can further increase the chances of a patient offering full, informed consent to treatment is to send them a copy of the consent form a few weeks before their proposed treatment date so they can digest it at their leisure and research anything of concern before the day of treatment. Never accept a pre-signed consent form, and never presume they have found the time to read it. Use it as a discussion point before beginning your own consent process in person.

## CONFLICT RESOLUTION

At some point or another, you are likely to either make a mistake or have a patient unhappy with the outcome of a treatment you have performed. Any complaints you receive will undoubtedly bring up strong emotions in you; however, you need to try to find out exactly *why* your patient is unhappy before coming up with a shared plan on how best to overcome this situation.

Should you encounter a complaint, the most important first step is to apologise to your patient. An apology is not an admission of guilt, nor does it mean that you agree with the nature of the complaint. The essence of an apology is demonstrating your ability to empathise with your patient that they are not happy with the treatment they have received. By apologising you are indicating to your patient that you understand their viewpoint, an essential step in deescalating a potential conflict.

It is strongly advisable to invite your patient into your clinic at the first possible opportunity. Body language and subtle nuances of language are important in expressing an emotional response which are only really achievable during a face-to-face discussion. Another important reason to see your patient in person is that you may well be able to easily rectify their grievance (such as lip asymmetry). Another reason why you should see your patient as soon as possible is that they may have a potentially dangerous complication which requires urgent medical attention. From an ethical perspective, it is strongly advisable to offer patients a review and treatment of complications free of charge, as it is wholly unethical to charge a patient for a complication you have inflicted on them.

When it comes to the meeting, take the time to ask them exactly what has happened and how it is upsetting them. Take the time to explore their ideas, concerns and expectations from a treatment. Try to start with open questions, such as *"What is it about your treatment you are unhappy with?"* Give them time to express what they are dissatisfied with and what they were initially expecting. A complaint may just be an expected finding which was not properly explained during the consenting process, such as swelling after lip augmentation with dermal fillers. If it is a recognised complication, then apologise again to your patient and offer them the potential strategies you could employ to rectify this. Let them make an informed decision about what strategy to employ next after giving them all the available information. Never attempt to simply placate your patients as it will make you sound disinterested and can further inflame the situation, be it real or perceived. If you are adequately trained and equipped to do so, then offer to treat any complications which have arisen. Be aware, however, that some people may not want the practitioner who caused a complication to treat them again. If this is the case, offer to refer them to an impartial second opinion as a matter of urgency.

Whenever you receive a serious complaint, ask your patient for consent to discuss what has happened with a trusted senior practitioner. If your patient consents to you doing so, then show the senior practitioner anonymised notes of your consultation and your pre- and post-procedure photographs to gain an impartial opinion on what has happened. It is often advisable to invite them to your consultation with your patient so they will be there as a second opinion on the day as well as for medicolegal protection should things escalate further.

Should your patient decline to meet you in person, then try to find out why without labouring the point or causing embarrassment. If they would prefer to see a different practitioner, then offer them the chance to see one; failing that, do your best to discuss things with them in any means you can.

If, despite your best attempts, you cannot resolve the conflict with your patient, then it is advisable to call your governing body and medicolegal team for advice. They will be able to offer your further help and support on the matter immediately as well as should, heaven forbid, if a legal challenge is made.

## DECLINING TO TREAT

Declining to treat a patient is a difficult situation to manage, and doing it tactfully is a skill which takes a long time to master. Patients will more often than not attend your clinics with the intention of receiving a particular treatment, and many of them will have been looking forward to them for months. You must therefore be able to broach this sensitive subject gently, as well as having sufficient rationale for declining to proceed with a treatment. A lack of evidence for your decision to decline to treat your patient will make it look like it is a subjective opinion as opposed to being evidence-based and in their best interests, hence why you should ensure you stay up-to-date with current literature to ensure you can counsel your patients to a high standard.

Reasons to not treat a patient can be divided into absolute contraindications and relative contraindications. In practice, it is the relative contraindications which cause you more grief as they are often harder to justify to a patient.

It is very rare to make the decision to not treat a patient immediately as they walk into your consultation room and usually will come after you have taken a full medical history and undertaken your physical assessment. Should a patient inform you they have an absolute contraindication, such as active tuberculosis, or should you notice a large facial abscess, then it is usually relatively easy to sensitively inform them that treatment would not be in their best interests as it could negatively impact their health. Most people will be understandable upon hearing this as they are unlikely to wish to risk their life for a cosmetic procedure which can be postponed.

Relative contraindications are far harder to explain to a patient and subsequently must be broached very sensitively. Start by exploring exactly which treatments your patient was after, why they wanted that particular treatment and what the overall cosmetic outcome they were after was. This approach may seem somewhat patronising, but it will help you gather more information about your patient's ideas and expectations from treatment. Relative contraindications are subjective to a practitioner performing any treatment, and sadly, they are a "grey area" in which there no absolute rights or wrongs. Remember you have a duty of care to your patient, and this may be the only time in your practice that a paternalistic approach is sensible or advisable.

---

**TABLE 7.2**

**Absolute and Relative Contraindications to Dermal Filler Treatment**

| Absolute Contraindication | Relative Contraindication |
|---|---|
| • Previous anaphylactic reaction to dermal fillers or lidocaine | • Immunosuppression (e.g. organ transplant patient) |
| • Active infection at the site of injection | • Dermal filler unlikely to deliver desired outcome/ likely to directly cause poor cosmesis |
| • Active infection local to the site of injection (e.g. dental abscess and lip augmentation) | • Recent aspirin/non-steroidal anti-inflammatory drug use |
| • Active systemic infection (e.g. urinary tract infection) | • Autoimmune disorders such as systemic lupus erythematosus or Hashimoto's thyroiditis |
| • Body dysmorphia | • Recent local facial piercing or dental work |
| • Coagulopathies/anticoagulant medication | • Keloid scarring |
| • Patient younger than age 18 | |

## TABLE 7.3
## Absolute and Relative Contraindications to Botulinum Toxin

| Absolute Contraindication | Relative Contraindication |
|---|---|
| • Previous anaphylactic reaction to botulinum toxin | • Patient currently taking any of the following: |
| • Previous anaphylactic reaction to albumin | • Aminoglycosides |
| • Active infection at the site of injection | • Penicillamine |
| • Active infection local to the site of injection (e.g. dental bacterial conjunctivitis and orbicularis oculi injection) | • Quinine |
| | • Chloroquine |
| | • Hydroxychloroquine |
| • Active systemic infection (e.g. urinary tract infection) | • Calcium channel blockers |
| • Myaesthenia gravis | • Aspirin/non-steroidal anti-inflammatory drugs |
| • Motor neurone disease | • Steroids |
| • Eaton-Lambert syndrome | • Low chance of successful outcome |
| • Pregnancy/breastfeeding | • Recent local facial piercing |
| • Body dysmorphia | |
| • Coagulopathies/anticoagulant medication | |
| • Patient younger than age 18 | |

Once you have ascertained your patient's level of understanding, take the time to carefully explain to them why you don't think treatment is in their best interest. One example may be a patient with static lines who believes botulinum toxin treatment will make them vanish and restore a youthful appearance. As a trained practitioner, you are well aware that this is not the case; however, your patient is not. It is inadvisable to bamboozle them with scientific jargon, so explain in plain English why the particular treatment will not work for them. It is often useful at this point to offer viable alternatives (if any) as your patient may not be aware that there is a more suitable treatment available.

# 8 Introduction to botulinum toxin

In the right hands, botulinum toxin is an effective treatment to treat dynamic lines and prevent static wrinkle formation. Although the preparation and administration of botulinum toxin is in itself a relatively simple undertaking, the science behind it is somewhat more complex. Understanding *how* botulinum toxin can be used to paralyse muscles in a targeted manner will allow you to use this potent neurotoxin in a safe and skilled way to the benefit of your patients.

## THE ANATOMY AND PHYSIOLOGY OF MOVEMENT

Movement is something so fantastically simple that we almost universally take it for granted and rarely consider the complex anatomy and physiological mechanisms involved in even the simplest motor functions. In this chapter, we discuss how botulinum toxin is able to inhibit movement to create a desired cosmetic outcome; however, before we can safely administer this drug, it is important to understand just how we move to appreciate its role in cosmesis.

### THE NERVE CELL

Neurons are made of a *cell body*, *dendrites* and an *axon*. Their basic function is to transmit electrical signals, or nerve impulses, from one part of the body to another. Due to the speed of electrical transmission, they are able to transfer information between cells incredibly quickly. The cell body of a neuron is where the nucleus is located, as well as organelles important in keeping the nerve cell alive such as the Golgi apparatus and mitochondria. Attached to the cell body are dendrites which receive neuronal impulses. Once an impulse is received, the cell body can then decide whether to transmit, propagate or dismiss an impulse, and one of the key determinants on which outcome occurs is the *strength* of the signal itself.

The axon is a long tubular structure which extends out of the cell body. The point of attachment to the cell body is known as the *axon hillock*, and it is at this point where an action potential is usually generated, a change in the polarisation of a neuron to allow propagation of a signal. The axon is surrounded by a myelin sheath which serves to insulate the axon and decrease the loss of electrical signal, similar to electrical cabling in your home. Neuronal impulses do not travel through the axon but skip along the outside of the myelin sheath between areas known as *nodes of Ranvier*. At the end of the axon is the axon terminal, a specialised region of finger-like projections which are in close proximity with *but not touching* another nerve or effector cells (such as muscle). See Figure 8.1.

DOI: 10.1201/9781003198840-8

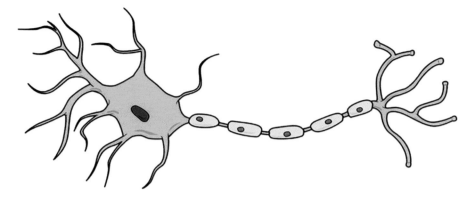

**FIGURE 8.1** Diagrammatic representation of a neuron.

The point at which a neuron interacts with another cell is known as a *synapse*. A synapse is a gap between axon terminals and the next cell, for example a dendrite of another neuron. A synapse is broken down into the *presynaptic terminal* of the cell conducting an electrical signal and a *postsynaptic terminal*, which is the region which receives said signal. There are two main types of synapse: *electrical* and *chemical* (Figure 8.2).

An electrical synapse occurs when the pre- and post-synaptic terminals are in electrical communication with one another. Ions are able to transfer between the synaptic terminals and subsequently these terminals are often bidirectional, allowing for signals to transfer back and forth. In some cases, there are *rectifying junctions*, which act as a one-way system for ions and subsequently regulate a unidirectional ion flow and synchronise the impulses of nerve cells. The transfer of nerve impulses along electrical synapses occurs almost immediately as the action of ion exchange is incredibly fast.

Chemical synapses rely on the secretion of *neurotransmitters* which diffuse along the synapse from the pre- to the post-synaptic membranes. Neurotransmitters are stored within synaptic vesicles which reside close to the cell membrane within the axon terminal of a neuron. When an action potential reaches the axon terminal, synaptic vesicles are stimulated to bind to the cell membrane and release their contents into the *synaptic cleft* – a term used to describe the gap between the pre- and post-synaptic membranes. Neurotransmitters diffuse across this cleft and bind to specific receptors on the cell membrane of the postsynaptic neuron.

As they require a diffusion gradient, chemical synapses are always unidirectional, as opposed to the previously described potentially bidirectional electrical synapses. Chemical synapses are wider than electrical synapses and are significantly slower in relaying a neuronal impulse. Depending on the neurotransmitter involved, chemical synapses can be further broken down into Type I *excitatory* synapses or Type II *inhibitory* synapses. Type I synapses are found on dendrites, whereas type II are found on cell bodies.

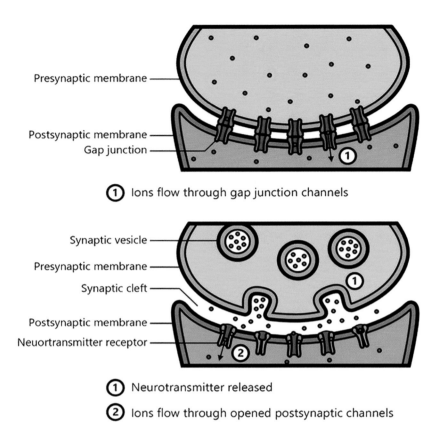

Presynaptic membrane

Postsynaptic membrane
Gap junction

(1) Ions flow through gap junction channels

Synaptic vesicle

Presynaptic membrane

Synaptic cleft

Postsynaptic membrane
Neuortransmitter receptor

(1) Neurotransmitter released
(2) Ions flow through opened postsynaptic channels

**FIGURE 8.2**   Electrical and chemical synapses.

There are over 50 described neurotransmitters, some of which are rapid-acting, such as glutamate and gamma aminobutyric acid, and others, such as growth hormone, function more slowly. As neurophysiology isn't the crux of this book, we shan't dwell too much on the slower-acting neurotransmitters; however, it is worth having an understanding of the rapidly acting transmitters, which can be reviewed in Table 8.1.

Of the neurotransmitters listed there, the one we are most interested in is acetylcholine, as botulinum toxin functions by inhibiting its release from the axon terminal at neuromuscular junctions.

Acetylcholine is utilised by neurons throughout the brain, such as in the motor cortex and in the motor neurons which innervate skeletal muscles. It has an almost universally excitatory effect; however, it has been detailed to be inhibitory at times at peripheral parasympathetic nerve endings, such as inducing bradycardia via the vagus nerve. It is also worth noting that acetylcholine is released from many sympathetic neurons, and subsequently, this is why botulinum toxin can also be used in the treatment of hyperhidrosis as sweating is a sympathetic response.

**TABLE 8.1**
**Small Molecule, Rapidly Acting Neurotransmitters**

| Class of Neurotransmitter | Examples |
|---|---|
| Class I | Acetylcholine |
| Class II (Amines) | Norepinephrine |
| | Epinephrine |
| | Dopamine |
| | Serotonin |
| | Histamine |
| Class III (Amino Acids) | Gamma-aminobutyric acid (GABA) |
| | Glycine |
| | Glutamate |
| | Aspartate |
| Class IV | Nitric oxide |

ANATOMY OF MOVEMENT

All conscious movements begin in a specialised area of the brain known as the *precentral gyrus* (Figure 8.3), which is colloquially known as the *motor strip*. The precentral gyrus is found in the posterior frontal lobe and is separated from the primary somatosensory cortex (the postcentral gyrus) by the central sulcus.

No matter which movement we are trying to initiate, the precentral gyrus is where it all begins. Within the precentral gyrus are neurons known as *Betz cells* that have long axons which course through the cerebral white matter. They progressively become closer to one another until they form part of the posterior limb of the internal capsule. Some of these fibres then travel to the opposite side of the brain where they synapse with the motor nuclei of the cranial nerves. These synapses can be found within the midbrain, pons and medulla oblongata. Those primary motor neurones which do not synapse with cranial nerves will continue inferiorly to the medulla oblongata, where the majority of them will cross the midline to the contralateral side. This is known as *pyramidal decussation.*

Once the primary motor neurones have exited the medulla oblongata inferiorly, they form the *anterior* and *posterior corticospinal tracts* (Figure 8.4). These tracts start in the cerebral cortex and travel through the spinal cord until they synapse with lower motor neurons responsible for trunk and limb movement. The anterior corticospinal tracts are made of primary motor neurons which do not decussate in the medulla oblongata and subsequently cross the midline in the spinal cord at the level they innervate. These tracts are responsible for the controlling movement of muscles of the trunk. The lateral corticospinal tracts make up more than 90% of the motor neurons within the spinal cord. Unlike the anterior corticospinal tracts, these tracts decussate within the medulla oblongata as opposed to the spinal cord. Due to this decussation, they innervate the contralateral side of the body from the cerebral hemisphere, which initiated a specific movement. The lateral corticospinal tracts are responsible for controlling the movement of the limbs and digits. Both the anterior and lateral corticospinal tracts synapse with lower motor neurons via the anterior horns of the spinal cord.

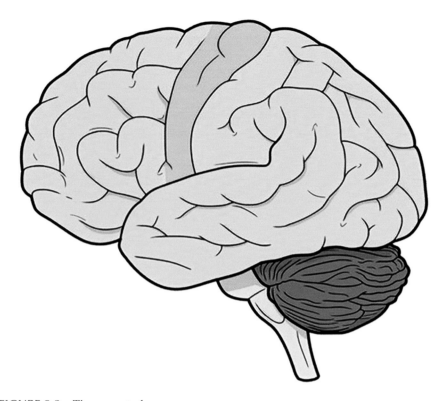

**FIGURE 8.3** The precentral gyrus.

## PHARMACOLOGY OF BOTULINUM TOXIN

Botulinum toxin is a proteolytic enzyme which functions by inhibiting the secretion of acetylcholine from afferent neurons at the neuromuscular junction. The toxin binds to the cell membrane of neurons which then form a vesicle around it to absorb it across the cell membrane through a process known as *endocytosis*. As the vesicle is taken through the cell membrane, the contents acidify, causing the vesicle to migrate further within the cell. Once the toxin is within the cytoplasm of an acetylcholine-secreting neurons, it cleaves *soluble NSF attachment protein receptors*, otherwise known as SNARE proteins. These proteins are essential in the *exocytosis* of vesicles and their contents from the presynaptic membrane into the presynaptic cleft. By irreversibly inhibiting the exocytosis of acetylcholine, botulinum toxin prevents neurons in the affected area from initiating movement at motor muscle endplates. In the realm of cosmetics, this prevents muscular movement and wrinkle formation.

Treatment with botulinum toxin causes a reversible chemical denervation at the level of the neuromuscular junction. This occurs via two distinct pathways; initially new, non-collateral axons grow on the affected neuron before a new, fully functional neuromuscular junction is developed at affected nerve terminals which replace the

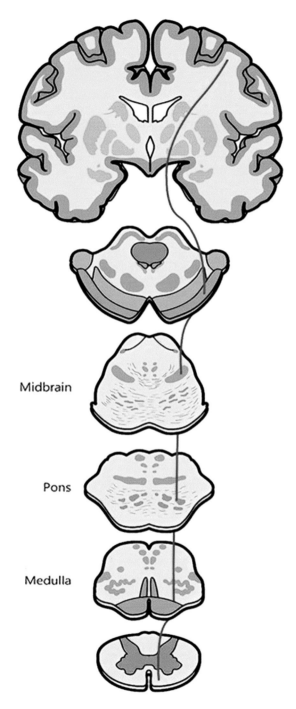

Midbrain

Pons

Medulla

**FIGURE 8.4** Corticospinal tracts.

original motor endplates. This process takes approximately 12 weeks from start to finish, which is reflective of the advised length of time a patient can experience paralysis due to botulinum toxin treatment.

Botulinum toxin is administered as an intramuscular injection and at recommended doses is believed to diffuse with a radius of approximately 1 cm from the injection site. As previously described, botulinum toxin causes partial chemical denervation of the injection site with resultant temporary muscle paralysis. There have been reports of subclinical weakness or muscle jitters at sites distant to where the toxin is administered, suggesting the toxin may spread via nerve axons or through the bloodstream. These symptoms are not dose-dependent and may occur after a solitary treatment; however, this has only been described in the literature in relation to medical-grade botulinum toxin used for the treatment of disorders such as cerebral palsy. Botulinum toxin is believed to be excreted via the liver in the proceeding weeks to months after treatment and there is no evidence to suggest it builds up within tissues.

## CONTRAINDICATIONS TO BOTULINUM TOXIN TREATMENT

In the right hands and with correct patient selection, botulinum toxin serves as an effective treatment for the prevention of static line formation. There are, however, a wide range of patients for whom this drug would not be safe for administration due to a risk of potentially serious side effects. Whenever you consent a patient for botulinum toxin treatment, you should screen them for potential contraindications to minimise the chance of causing them harm (Table 8.2).

---

### TABLE 8.2
### Contraindications to Botulinum Toxin Treatment

| Absolute Contraindication | Relative Contraindication |
|---|---|
| • Previous anaphylactic reaction to botulinum toxin | • Patient currently taking |
| • Previous anaphylactic reaction to albumin |   • Aminoglycosides |
| • Active infection at the site of injection |   • Penicillamine |
| • Active infection local to the site of injection (e.g. dental bacterial conjunctivitis and orbicularis oculi injection) |   • Quinine |
| • Active systemic infection (e.g. urinary tract infection) |   • Chloroquine |
| • Myaesthenia gravis |   • Hydroxychloroquine |
| • Motor neuron diseases |   • Calcium Channel blockers |
| • Eaton-Lambert syndrome |   • Aspirin |
| • Pregnancy/breastfeeding |   • Non-steroidal anti-inflammatory drugs |
| • Body dysmorphia |   • Steroids |
| • Coagulopathies/anticoagulant medication | • Botulinum toxin unlikely to deliver desired outcome/likely to cause poor cosmesis |
| • Patient younger than age 18 | • Recent local facial piercing |

Whenever you take a history before treating a patient with botulinum toxin, ensure that you ask specifically about all the mentioned contraindications. Although some listed are only relative contraindications, best practices dictate that it is safest to avoid treating these patients altogether as the risk of treatment is likely to outweigh the benefit.

**TABLE 8.3**

**Symptoms of Common Neuromuscular Conditions**

| Condition | Common Symptoms |
|---|---|
| Myasthenia gravis (MG) | Muscle weakness of specific muscle groups which is worse when tired and relieves with rest. Predominantly occurs in women younger than 40 years old and men older than 60 Common symptoms include the following: <ul><li>Drooping eyelids</li><li>Double vision</li><li>Difficulty chewing and swallowing</li><li>Difficulty speaking/hoarse or quiet voice</li><li>Difficulty walking</li><li>Fatigue</li></ul> Of note, in MG the legs are commonly more severely affected than the arms |
| Motor neuron diseases (MND) | Umbrella term for a plethora of similar conditions. Usually slow-onset muscle weakness May present as a child or later in life Three main patterns have been described: <ul><li>Asymmetrical distal weakness</li><li>Symmetrical muscle weakness</li><li>Symmetrical, focal, midline muscle weakness</li></ul> Sensory loss is not a common symptom of MND. There may be an associated family history. Other pertinent symptoms include the following: <ul><li>Fatigue</li><li>Muscle wasting</li><li>Difficulty chewing and swallowing</li><li>Clumsiness or altered gait</li></ul> |
| Eaton-Lambert syndrome | Usually occurs in patients older than age 40 Common symptoms include the following: <ul><li>Primarily proximal muscle weakness, relieved by exercise</li><li>Weakness worsened by high temperatures</li><li>Autonomic nervous system dysfunction: dry mouth/constipation/blurred vision/decreased sweating/orthostatic hypotension</li><li>Difficulty swallowing</li><li>Eye muscle weakness is uncommon.</li></ul> |

One key concern regarding treatment with botulinum toxin is that your patients may not have been formally diagnosed with a contraindicated condition. It will become clearly apparent from your initial medical consultation if a patient is aged younger than 18 or if they are taking medications which prevent botulinum toxin treatment, yet an insidious condition may not be clearly apparent to you or them at the time of consultation. It is therefore worth asking about the following symptoms which may indicate an underlying neuromuscular condition.

Should you see a patient who exhibits any of the symptoms in Table 8.3, then it is strongly advisable to not treat them and advise them to see their general practitioner. It is inadvisable to try to diagnose them in the setting of a cosmetic clinic; however, they probably would warrant further assessment by a neurologist to explore their symptoms further.

# 9 Botulinum toxin practical skills

Once you have garnered a solid theoretical understanding of the relevant anatomy and physiology of botulinum toxin treatment, as well as the underlying pharmacology of the drug, you will be able to safely administer this treatment for dynamic lines. In this chapter, we discuss ways in which you can treat the three most commonly treated areas with botulinum toxin: the frontalis muscles, glabellar complex and orbicularis oculi muscles.

## RECONSTITUTION OF BOTULINUM TOXIN

Botulinum toxin should be dissolved in saline pre-administration. Either bacteriostatic or normal saline are suitable for reconstitution; however, patients often report that botulinum toxin reconstituted with bacteriostatic saline is less painful and more tolerable when administered in comparison to normal saline. It is worth noting that you should not use water for injection to dilute botulinum toxin as it not only is more painful but also confers a risk of tissue necrosis. Once you have reconstituted your botulinum toxin, gently swirl the contents of the vial in a circular motion to ensure they have dissolved sufficiently before injecting your patient. Your chosen brand of botulinum toxin will be able to advise you on the volume of saline to use for reconstitution. Once reconstituted, it is advisable to keep it refrigerated and use your toxin within four hours; however, some studies suggest it will retain its potency for up to six weeks after reconstitution as long as it is kept refrigerated between 2°C–8°C.

## ASEPTIC NON-TOUCH TECHNIQUE

There are two forms of asepsis used in health care: *surgical* and *medical*. The key difference between these two strategies to minimise infection is that in surgical asepsis, the intention is to *remove* microorganisms from an area such as an operating theatre, whereas medical asepsis focuses on *minimising* the number and preventing the spread of microorganisms. Surgical asepsis is essentially a sterile technique, utilising technology such as the use of laminar flow in orthopaedic surgery. It is not practical to create or maintain surgical asepsis outside of a designated operating theatre, and subsequently the vast majority of clinic-based cosmetic procedures are practised under medical asepsis.

The most common form of medical asepsis in clinical practice is the *aseptic non-touch technique* (ASNTT), which focuses on preventing microorganisms

DOI: 10.1201/9781003198840-9

from the practitioner or patient reaching critical sites, for example, preventing any bacteria on your hands being unwittingly introduced into your patient. ASNTT has a few underlying key concepts, such as *key parts*, *key sites* and an *aseptic field*.

Key parts are parts of your equipment which must remain sterile and avoid microbial contamination, such as your needle, the connecting portion of needle and syringe and the contents of your vials of botulinum toxin and saline for reconstitution. The key site in question with cosmesis is the area of skin treated, and the creation of an aseptic field here will further decrease the odds of bacterial contamination. An aseptic field can be created by disinfecting an area and covering the surrounding skin with a sterile covering, only allowing the area to be treated to be exposed. It is best practice to avoid touching this area unless absolutely critical, and in the realms of cosmesis, you will likely need to place your fingers in close proximity to the key area to anchor the skin or introduce treatments. It is advisable, therefore, that you use sterile gloves when touching or manipulating a key area. The mouth is a difficult place to maintain asepsis, as despite your best efforts, the mouth is home to millions of bacteria, and it is almost impossible to prevent any of these from migrating to the treatment area, such as when performing lip augmentation. It is crucial, however, that you do your utmost to maintain sterility regardless.

The first step in the ASNTT is to perform a thorough hand-washing through the World Health Organization–advised seven-step technique with warm, soapy water. Once you have washed your hands, it is imperative you do not touch anything else apart from sterile paper towels and sterile gloves. Once you are wearing sterile gloves you can only maintain sterility if you endeavour to only touch other sterile equipment until they have been removed.

The seven-step handwashing technique is as follows:

1. Rinse your hands under warm water and place a fifty-pence size piece of soap in the palm of either hand before rubbing your palms together
2. Rub the back of both hands
3. Interlace your fingers and rub your hands together with your palms facing each other
4. Interlace your fingers and rub the back of each hand with the palm of the other hand
5. Clean the thumb and each finger of both hands individually with the other hand
6. Rub the palm with the fingers of the other hand
7. Clasp the wrist and clean this area last

Once you have washed your hands, use a sterile paper towel to dab them dry, as vigorous drying in a rubbing motion can exfoliate the skin and expose foreign bodies and microorganisms, subsequently desterilising the area.

Once you have cleaned your hands, you can adhere to the ASNTT through the following steps:

- Clean your work surfaces with a disinfectant wipe or spray with disinfectant and wipe with a sterile paper towel.
- Open your wound pack whilst only touching the corners, allowing the central portion to remain sterile.
- Open the packaging and drop your essential equipment into your newly created sterile field.
- Wash your hands again, put on sterile gloves and clean the key area of your patient with a sterilising swab.
- Cover the key area with a sterile drape.
- Wash your hands and put on sterile gloves once more.
- Perform your treatment, taking care to minimise contact with the key area and avoiding touching key parts.

Once you have performed your treatment, place all used equipment in sharps bins or clinical waste bins as necessary. Clean your work surfaces with disinfectant wipes or spray and wash your hands once more.

## SKIN PREPARATION FOR BOTULINUM TOXIN ADMINISTRATION

Take care to appropriately sterilise the region you intend to treat. Alcohol swabs are usually sufficient, but they may cause skin irritation or dryness. Ensure that all makeup has been removed from the area with your initial cleaning, before cleaning the area from the region of treatment again. Do not scrub the area, but instead, clean in a firm unidirectional continuous motion. Dispose of your swabs as clinical waste. Once you have prepared the area, let the skin air-dry for approximately one minute before starting your injections. Although it is impractical to administer botulinum toxin without touching the area after sterilisation, try to minimise any contact you may make with the skin to minimise infection risk. It is also worth only using sterile gloves during the procedure to further reduce the risk of introducing infection.

## ADMINISTRATION OF BOTULINUM TOXIN

Botulinum toxin is an intramuscular injection; therefore, failure to deliver it into the muscle will make a desirable cosmetic outcome unlikely. As with most intramuscular injections, you should administer your needle at ninety degrees to the skin (see Figure 9.1). Once you become a bit more experienced with injecting into the relatively superficial muscles of the face you will develop a good appreciation for how the epidermis, dermis, subcutaneous tissues and muscle feel as you introduce the needle. Be careful when advancing the needle as should it penetrate too far, then you

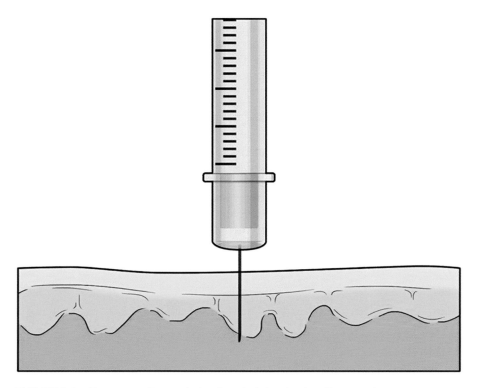

**FIGURE 9.1**    Correct needle angulation for administering botulinum toxin.

may strike the periosteum of the underlying bone, which will be exquisitely painful for your patient.

Pain during toxin administration is multifactorial but can be minimised with good injection technique and appropriate equipment. As detailed earlier, the use of bacteriostatic saline will make the injection more tolerable. Another potential cause of pain is the calibre of your needle, so use the smallest diameter needle available to you (try to avoid using a needle larger than 26G to decrease discomfort). One final consideration is the pain caused by hydrodistension of tissues when you inject. Although injecting a volume of fluid is necessary for treatment, injecting slowly and to the correct depth will lessen the discomfort felt by your patient. Due to the increased hydrostatic pressure whilst administering the solution, try to use the minimum required volume to create the desired cosmesis to decrease the amount of tissue stretching and pain associated with this.

## FRONTALIS

As discussed in our anatomy chapter, the frontalis is a wide, flat muscle which runs the along the anterior aspect of the forehead. The frontalis is the primary elevator of the eyebrows and is primarily responsible for forehead wrinkles, which is why it is a frequently targeted site for botulinum toxin treatment (Figure 9.2).

Standard practice for treating the frontalis muscle is to administer four injections in a horizontal line across the forehead. Never inject lateral to the mid-pupillary line due to risk of accidentally paralysing the temporalis muscles which confers an increased risk of ptosis and/or eyebrow drooping. There are two schools of thought regarding where you should administer your toxin, and neither is incorrect. You may choose to assess where the greatest amount of forehead wrinkling is on raising the eyebrows and inject in a line across that site. The other technique you may wish to employ is to calculate the midline between the eyebrows and the hairline and inject horizontally along there.

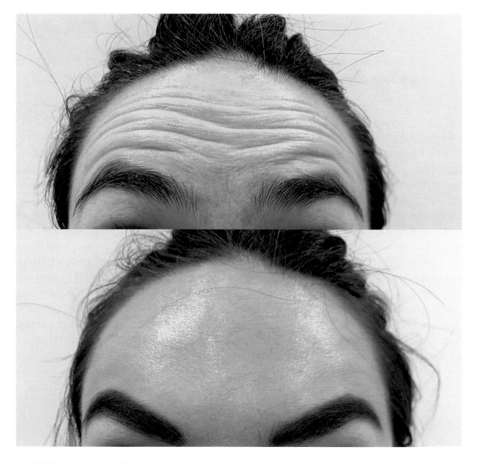

FIGURE 9.2    The effects of botulinum toxin on the frontalis muscle.

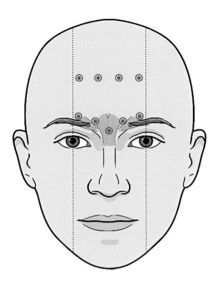

**FIGURE 9.3**   Advised injection sites to treat the frontalis muscle and glabella complex.

The forehead contains very little subcutaneous fat and your injection into the muscle will rarely be more than a few millimetres deep. Due to this, it is very easy to strike periosteum and cause your patient discomfort, so be careful when introducing your needle. Inject perpendicular to the skin and administer the advised dose. Once injected, place firm sustained pressure over the injection sites (Figure 9.3) to decrease the risk of bruising and to ensure adequate haemostasis.

As the frontalis is a large muscle and there being minimal surface anatomy to rely on, you may find that wrinkles form in the areas you have not treated by the time you review your patients. This is not a major problem and is easily rectified by performing targeted injections on your review appointment. Consider using the same dose as your initial treatment where required to rectify this. Advise your patients they may notice a few new wrinkles due to the skin ruffling at a new site when attempting to move the eyebrows so that they are not taken aback by this in the interim. One useful trick to decrease the formation of lumps akin to beestings after administering botox is to place a fresh piece of gauze along the forehead and apply gentle, sustained pressure for a minute or so once you have finished the treatment. This often decreases the prominence of these unsightly bumps and decreases the changes of bruises forming.

## GLABELLAR COMPLEX

At the time of writing, the glabellar complex is the only region of the face in which botulinum toxin is licenced for cosmetic use. The glabellar complex is a relatively strong group of muscles, responsible for pulling the eyebrows in an inferomedial direction allowing us to frown, which, in turn, creates wrinkles in this region (Figure 9.4).

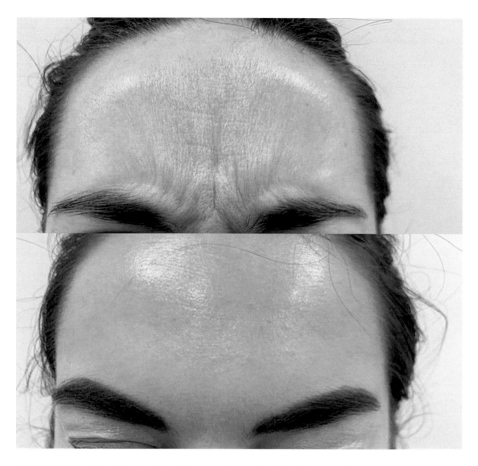

**FIGURE 9.4** The effects of botulinum toxin on the glabellar complex.

As with the frontalis muscle, the glabellar complex is treated with a series of injections perpendicular to the skin (Figure 9.5). It usually comprises five injections; the medial three are usually each double the dose of the most lateral two. When injecting the glabellar complex, start with the procerus muscle which is found just superior to the bridge of the nose. Ask your patient to frown as much as they can. Whilst they are frowning, pinch the belly of the procerus muscle between your thumb and index finger as this will be your target for injecting. Treating the procerus will most likely be the deepest injection you administer for botulinum toxin, and you may need to go down to the hilt of the needle.

Once you have treated the procerus, the corrugators are relatively easy muscles to treat. Yet again, inject with your needle inserted at ninety degrees to the skin. Your injection site for the corrugators should be approximately 1 cm above the bony orbital margin, so ensure you palpate this area before choosing your target site. One useful technique is to rest your index finger horizontally on the bony orbital rim whilst

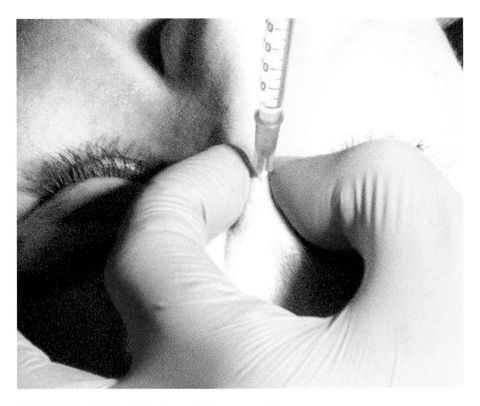

**FIGURE 9.5**    Advised injection technique to treat the procerus.

injecting to ensure you are in the correct location and to decrease the chance of
the toxin spreading inferiorly. Inferior spread of botulinum toxin may inadvertently
paralyse the levator palpebrae superioris muscles, resulting in an eyelid droop. After
injecting, keep your finger rested on top of the orbital rim for approximately thirty
seconds to further decrease the chances of the toxin spreading inferiorly (Figure 9.6).

    One key caution to consider when injecting the glabellar complex is that the supe-
rior orbital nerve runs superiorly from the supraorbital notch towards the hairline.
This nerve is not infrequently damaged by injectors as it can be difficult to be certain
of its route, so it is essential you consent your patients for neuropraxia or neuralgia
due to botulinum toxin therapy.

## CROW'S FEET

*Crow's feet* is a colloquial term used in reference to wrinkles caused by the orbicularis oculi muscles, and these wrinkles are usually most noticeable when a person
smiles or squints (Figure 9.7).

    When treating this area, yet again take note to palpate your injection site a mini-
mum of 1cm from the lateral bony orbital rim. It is useful to use your finger as both

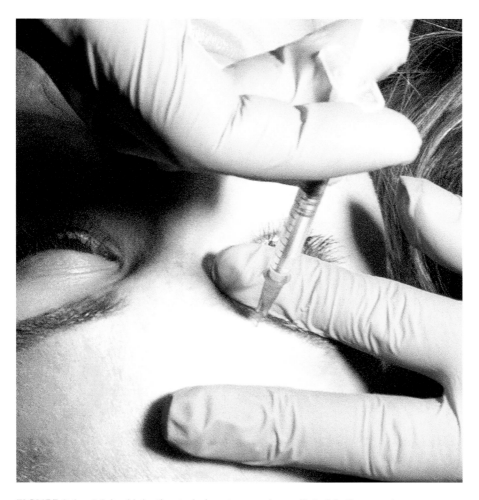

**FIGURE 9.6** Advised injection technique to treat the medial glabellar complex.

a marker and barrier against toxin spread when injecting as you would when treating the glabella complex. Three injections are used for each side when treating the orbicularis oculi muscle with the middle injection ever so slightly lateral to the others (Figure 9.8). It is best practice to treat the orbicularis oculi muscle with the patient lying flat so as to decrease the chance of botulinum toxin spreading medially into the levator palpebrae muscles. This risk is further mitigated by leaving your finger in place for 30 seconds after toxin injection to decrease the risk of it spreading medially.

You may find that the orbicularis oculi muscles are surprisingly deep and that you need to introduce your needle to the hilt. As always, introduce your needle slowly and carefully to decrease the risk of striking the periosteum. One of the main reasons that treating this area fails is simply because practitioners are too fearful when

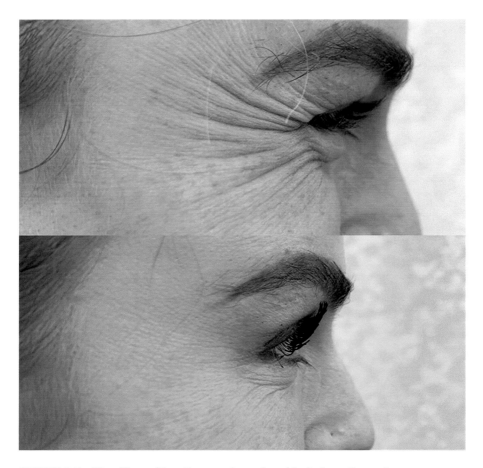

FIGURE 9.7    The effects of botulinum toxin on the orbicularis oculi muscles.

introducing their needle and accidentally deliver the botulinum toxin into subcutaneous fat as opposed to the desired muscle layer.

## AFTERCARE

After treatment with botulinum toxin it is advisable to tell your patients to relax for
the rest of the day. To ensure the best cosmetic outcomes and to decrease the risk of
complications, advise your patients to avoid the following:

- Wearing make-up on the treated area for the rest of the day
- Lying flat for four hours post-treatment
- Vigorous washing of the area or exfoliation
- Extremes of temperature (hot or cold)
- Anything which makes them hot and sweaty

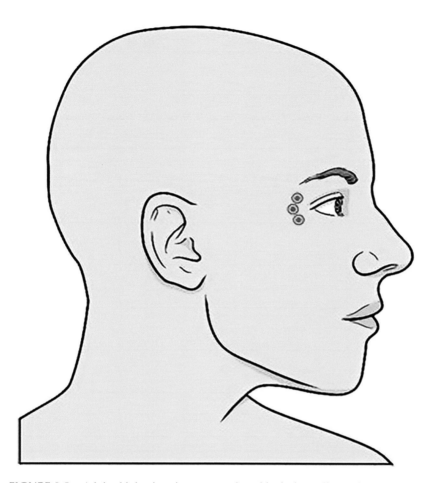

**FIGURE 9.8** Advised injection sites to treat the orbicularis oculi muscles.

- Saunas/steam rooms
- Alcohol
- Sunbeds

The reason for avoiding alcohol or becoming hot and sweaty in any capacity is due to the theoretical risk that vasodilation will potentiate toxin spread and risk inadvertently paralysing the wrong muscle groups, as is the case for alcohol. Lying flat or rubbing the face will potentially allow toxin to spread into other compartments mechanically. Make-up and steam rooms are risk factors for post-procedure infection.

Some practitioners advise patients to move the treated area as much as possible in the hours after treatments to allow the toxin to "*work its way in*". You may choose to advise this or not as there is no evidence it is beneficial, nor is there evidence that it is not.

Always arrange for a review two weeks after botulinum toxin treatment. This will allow you to see your patient and address any new dynamic lines which have formed, as well as ensure that there is an acceptable cosmetic outcome from your initial treatment. The minimum two-week timescale is worth adhering to religiously (unless there has been a complication which requires rectification sooner) as after two weeks the effects of botulinum toxin should be visible and unlikely to change acutely. Treat any areas of undesirable movement (sticking to the same rules as before) with the advised dose of toxin from your supplier. The two-week review is not only useful in ensuring cosmesis but also for you to be able to keep an eye on your patient to intercept any potential evolving complications.

Table 9.1 gives a concordance of product details.

**TABLE 9.1**
**Examples of Common Botulinum Toxin Preparations**

| Product Name | Toxin | Manufacturer |
| --- | --- | --- |
| Botox | Onobotulinumtoxin A | Allergan |
| Vistabel | Onobotulinumtoxin A | Allergan |
| Dysport | Abobotulinumtoxin A | Ipsen |
| Azzalure | Abobotulinumtoxin A | Ipsen |
| Xeomin | Incobotulinumtoxin A | Merz |
| Bocouture | Incobotulinumtoxin A | Merz |
| Jeuveau | Prabobotulinumtoxin A | Evolus |

# 10 Botulinum toxin complications and management

Risks are conferred whenever you undertake an intervention on a patient, with varying degrees of severity. It is imperative that you do not undertake a treatment unless you are competent and confident to rectify any complications you may incur. There is no way a risk can be entirely eliminated; however, you should make every effort to minimise the risk of any potential complications and be aware of their manifestations to allow for prompt treatment. In this chapter, we outline some of the more common complications of botulinum toxin treatment and some approaches you may wish to take to address them should they occur. This is by no means an exhaustive list, and management guidelines are frequently updated, so it is strongly advisable to continually refresh and supplement your knowledge with the most up-to-date literature. Anaphylaxis is a potential risk of botulinum toxin treatment; its management is discussed in the later chapter regarding complications of dermal filler augmentation.

## SYSTEMIC SPREAD OF TOXIN

Botulinum toxin is one of the most potent neuromuscular inhibitors on the planet and it as previously discussed its discovery was linked to the disease *botulism*, a potentially fatal condition. Botulism is characterised by weakness, fatigue, blurred vision, dysphagia, incontinence, respiratory distress, dysarthria and potentially death. Paralysis secondary to botulism may last for up to two months, and if untreated up to half of those affected die of the disease. Even if treated, between up to one in 10 patients who contract botulism die. The treatment of botulism involves administering botulinum antitoxin and supportive care such as mechanical ventilation.

In cosmetic practice, systemic spread of toxin is a very rare complication, but you must still consent your patients for it as previously discussed. Botulinum toxin has approximately a 1-cm radius of diffusion when injected intramuscularly and is unlikely to extravasate into the systemic circulation. When used therapeutically for spasticity disorders, long-term weakness has been reported in a handful of prospective cohort studies, as well as approximately a one in 100 chance of urinary incontinence and admission to hospital with respiratory symptoms, such as difficulty breathing.

Take the time to consent your patients of the early signs of systemic spread of botulinum toxin, advising them to seek urgent medical attention should they develop speech disturbances, swallowing, urinary or respiratory problems shortly after administration. Advise your patients to go straight to hospital should they develop

DOI: 10.1201/9781003198840-10

these symptoms, as arranging to see you (unless you have a fully staffed intensive care unit and sufficient quantities of botulinum antitoxin) will not only waste valuable time but will likely prove to be fruitless. When advising your patients to attend hospital ensure that they do not drive themselves, as the risk of muscle paralysis and loss of consciousness are significant in this instance – adding the potential risks of harm to themselves or others in a road traffic collision. Instead, suggest they call for an emergency ambulance or, if able and safe to do so, get a relative or friend to drive them to hospital as a matter of urgency.

It is also imperative to inform your patients of the potential long-term sequelae of systemic spread. Inform them that subjective long-term weakness may present itself several months after botulinum toxin therapy; however, in the majority of cases, it will resolve spontaneously.

The risk of systemic spread of toxin can be mitigated by adhering to the advised dosage units of your choice of botulinum toxin, having a good understanding of the relevant surface anatomy of your treatment areas and only using advised injection techniques.

## CELLULITIS

Cellulitis is an infection of the dermis and subcutaneous fat of the skin. Clinically it will present as a localised spreading, erythematous area which is warm and tender to touch. If untreated, it may become severe enough to cause systemic upset (pyrexia, general malaise, etc.) and potentially more serious sequelae such as abscess formation or sepsis.

Cellulitis is usually bacterial in origin and the primary causative organisms are skin commensals such as Group A *Streptococcus* and *Staphylococcus aureus* which enter the skin via defects, such as a cut or an abrasion. In the context of cosmetic procedures, it is invariably introduced via inadequate sterilisation of the tissues or improper sterile technique when administering fillers or botulinum toxin.

When examining a patient with suspected cellulitis, check for needle marks from where you may have administered botulinum toxin and see if the tender, erythematous area relates to your area of treatment. Injecting botulinum toxin in the forehead is unlikely to result in cellulitis of the leg; however, an area of erythema adjacent to where you administered botulinum toxin to treat the glabellar complex should raise clinical suspicion.

Your patient will likely present with an area of hot, red and exquisitely tender skin. The afflicted area will likely look tight and shiny, with or without overlying dry patches. Should the cellulitis be inadequately treated, then tissues will become indurated and firmer to the touch as the infection progresses.

When palpating the area, try to ensure you cannot feel a fluctuant mass, as this may be more likely to represent an abscess formation which will require different definitive management, as discussed in Chapter 13. In reality, as botulinum toxin is diluted primarily with normal or bacteriostatic saline, abscess formation is much less likely than with dermal fillers. This is because the constituents of dermal filler (such as glycosaminoglycans) can be metabolised by microorganisms as well as offering pathogens a protective buffer from the immune system. Due to the beneficial effects of dermal filler in propagating microbiota, failure to create sufficient asepsis can result in bacteria being introduced to the dermal layer with all the requisite materials to form a deep-seated infection and resultant abscess formation.

Before you begin treating an area of cellulitis, first, assess the patient's observations to ensure they are not clinically septic and require hospital admission. Mark around the edge of the affected area with a permanent marker, as this will allow you and your patient to assess whether the area of infection is progressing or resolving with therapy. A common first-line antibiotic choice is flucloxacillin 500 mg four times daily for 7 days, provided the patient is not penicillin-allergic, nor do they require dose adjustments or have any other contraindications. If your patient is penicillin-allergic, then you may consider using clindamycin or clarithromycin. Ensure you review your patient daily and take a full set of observations to check that the infection is not spreading, an abscess is not forming, and that they are not becoming septic. Should the infection not resolve with empirical antibiotic therapy, then you should refer them to secondary care for further assessment and management. It is advisable to write a letter for them to take with them for the secondary care physicians outlining which cosmetic procedures you have performed (dates, product, volume), as well as the management you have administered thus far. Ensure you also contact your product manufacturer with the batch number of the product you used, as an investigation should be mounted to assess whether the entire batch of botulinum toxin or saline is infected or if yours is an isolated case.

When considering cellulitis in the context of botulinum toxin therapy, especially regarding the glabellar complex and orbicularis oculi muscles, you must be aware of orbital and periorbital cellulitis as these require urgent specialist attention.

## ORBITAL AND PERIORBITAL CELLULITIS

Both orbital and periorbital cellulitis may be caused by tracking infection of the soft tissues surrounding the orbit. Should the infection make its way to the eye itself then, there the consequences can be devastating. The key anatomical discriminator for orbital or periorbital cellulitis is the *orbital septum*, a thin, fibrous, multilaminated structure which attaches peripherally to the orbital margin to form the *arcus marginalis* which provides mechanical support to the orbital fat. Should an infection remain anterior to the orbital septum then this is known as *periorbital cellulitis*, whereas should it penetrate the septum and enter the soft tissues within the orbit, it is known as *orbital cellulitis*.

## PERIORBITAL CELLULITIS

Periorbital cellulitis (otherwise known as preseptal cellulitis) is the less severe of these two conditions as the inflammatory process involves the superficial periorbital soft tissues *without* involving the globe or orbit. Despite having a better prognosis than orbital cellulitis, periorbital cellulitis still necessitates swift diagnosis and management to decrease morbidity.

Common presenting features of periorbital cellulitis are oedema and erythema of the eyelid and soft tissues surrounding the eye. Secondary signs may also include conjunctival injection, low-grade fever and difficulty opening the eyelids. As peri-orbital cellulitis does not invade the orbit, patients do not have visual impairment, proptosis, or limited or painful eye movements. This can only be ascertained with a prompt and detailed ophthalmic examination.

The likely causative organisms in periorbital cellulitis are *Staphyloccus aureus* and *Streptococcus spp.* Historically, *Haemophilus influenzae* type B was a promi-nent cause; however, most people in the United Kingdom are now vaccinated against this particular pathogen. If your patient has a fever or is clinically septic, is immu-nocompromised or if you are unable to assess the eye due to swelling, then you should admit them to hospital as an emergency. Co-amoxiclav or Clindamycin are sensible antibiotic choices for mild periorbital cellulitis, and these patients may be managed as an outpatient. If you are appropriately trained and competent to do so, review them daily for the next few days to ensure they are improving. Should they be unable to attend for daily review, fail to improve or should their symptoms worsen, then refer them urgently to hospital where they may require intravenous antibiotic treatment. When referring your patient, write a letter to the admitting doctor for the patient to take with them, outlining the dates of treatment, product used, and your examination findings.

### ORBITAL CELLULITIS

Should a tracking cellulitis penetrate the orbital septum then there is a strong pos-sibility the patient will develop orbital cellulitis. Accurate diagnosis and treatment of orbital cellulitis is crucial in preventing serious consequences such as optic neu-ropathy, encephalomeningitis, cavernous sinus thrombosis, sepsis and intracranial abscess formation.

Orbital cellulitis will present with localised oedema and erythema in the soft tis-sues surrounding the eye similar to periorbital cellulitis. Key discriminating factors which should make you consider orbital cellulitis as a likely diagnosis is proptosis, ophthalmoplegia, decreased visual acuity (and colour vision) and painful eye move-ments. In severe cases, patients may have a relative afferent pupillary defect or pres-ent with symptoms of stroke or encephalitis. Should a patient present with any of these symptoms, also take the time to take a full set of observations including their neurological status. Please note, following botulinum toxin therapy, should a patient present with an isolated ophthalmoplegia, then this may be due to misadministration of toxin as opposed to an underlying infection.

Causative organisms for orbital cellulitis are unsurprisingly similar to those for periorbital cellulitis, with *Staphylococcus aureus*, *Streptococcus pyogenes* and *Haemophilus influenzae* type B being the three most likely pathogens. Despite hav-ing similar causative organisms, oral antibiotics are unlikely to be effective in treat-ing orbital cellulitis, and this is a condition you should *not* attempt to treat in the community.

If you suspect a patient has orbital cellulitis, stay with them whilst you arrange for an urgent assessment in eye casualty by the on-call ophthalmologist (Table 10.1). If you are unable to get through to them, write a letter of your treatment dates and

**TABLE 10.1**
**Ophthalmic Signs in Periorbital and Orbital Cellulitis**

| Sign | Periorbital Cellulitis | Orbital Cellulitis |
|------|------------------------|--------------------|
| Proptosis | No | Yes |
| Eye movements | Normal | Limited, painful |
| Visual acuity | Normal | Decreased |
| Colour vision | Normal | Decreased |
| Relative afferent pupillary defect | No | Yes |

products used for the patient to take to accident and emergency. They are unlikely to be safe to drive so ensure they have a safe way to get to the hospital. Treatment of orbital cellulitis is usually in the form of intravenous antibiotics (such as Tazocin) with a minimum of four-hourly ophthalmological and neurological examinations. Most patients will require a CT scan on admission to assess for any intra-orbital collection or intracranial abscesses. Should there be an orbital collection, patients usually require surgery to evacuate this.

## EYEBROW ASYMMETRY

Eyebrow asymmetry is one of the most common complications following botulinum toxin treatment. It is frequently caused by under-treating the glabellar complex or the frontalis. Should the glabellar be under-treated, then the eyebrow will appear raised on that particular side; conversely, if you were to under-treat the frontalis, then that eyebrow will be depressed and medialised on the side of treatment.

Eyebrow asymmetry is one of the main reasons why it is best practice to review all your botulinum toxin patients after two weeks. The effects of toxin should be noticeable by this point and will allow you to objectively assess the region requiring further treatment. Fixing eyebrow asymmetry is usually straightforward in the majority of cases simply by administrating further toxin in the under-treated area.

The risk of eyebrow asymmetry is much lower if you understand the relevant anatomy; however, it still may be difficult to be able to accurately predict the true location of both the frontalis muscle and glabellar complex. Consent your patients to this potential complication prior to starting treatment and reassure them at the time of the initial consultation that should it present it is usually remedied with relative ease.

Some patients have persistent eyebrow asymmetry despite your best efforts at follow-up. In this instance, you will have two options: to do something or to do nothing. It may be worth attempting a further treatment in the under-treated area; however, if it wasn't effective previously, there are no guarantees it will be effective a second time. This may mean you are injecting a patient and inflicting pain and a risk of complications with no benefit. The other is to counsel your patient that the botulinum toxin effects should wear off over the next three to four months and therefore the undesired cosmesis will spontaneously resolve.

## TREATING THE WRONG AREA

Before starting your cosmetic practice, it is essential to understand the surface anatomy of the face to decrease the chance of accidentally treating the wrong area and conferring morbidity on your patients. In saying that, the anatomy of every patient you see will be slightly different, and it is almost impossible to know for certain that you are injecting the correct muscle group. Common areas which are inadvertently treated are the zygomaticus major muscle when treating the orbicularis oculi muscle as well as accidentally injecting the temporalis muscle when treating the frontalis.

Due to the delay from treatment to muscle paralysis in botulinum toxin therapy, you are unlikely to know for sure that you have treated the wrong area at the time of injecting. Should a patient report an inability to smile or move the ipsilateral side of the face from day one post-treatment of the orbicularis oris muscle, then it is likely your toxin has been delivered to the wrong area. If a patient reports this to you, then arrange for an urgent review to assess it further. Ensure that the patient has only lower motor neuron signs *in the affected area*, as a Bell's palsy or stroke could be a confounding diagnosis. If your patient has any upper motor neuron symptoms or if their symptoms are progressing, then make arrangements for an urgent medical assessment in secondary care.

If it transpires that it is a simple case of injecting the wrong area, then apologise to your patient and admit that it is likely due to the botulinum toxin administration. You have a duty of candour to your patients, and it is imperative that you are honest in this situation. Advise them that the symptoms are likely to last for three to four months as with any other area treated with botulinum toxin.

## NEUROPRAXIA AND NEURALGIA

Neuropraxia and neuralgia are infrequent complications of botulinum toxin therapy and are primarily caused by incorrect needle placement. As we discussed in our anatomy chapter, the superior orbital nerve tracks superiorly from the superior orbital notch. It passes upwards underneath the lateral aspect of the corrugator and frontalis muscles towards the scalp. Due to the close proximity of these nerves, as you insert your needle to treat these areas there is a chance you may accidentally traumatise them.

Should you hit the supraorbital nerve, the patient will likely report immediate, terrible pain shooting up to their scalp at the time of injection. This neuralgia will be intense and similar to *brain freeze*, which we have all encountered at some point eating a cold ice cream. This pain may remain for several days to weeks before resolution due to the slow rate of healing of peripheral nerves. Advise your patients to take sufficient analgesia during this time and reassure them it should settle over due course. Most of the time the symptoms are brought by *brushing* the nerve; however, research suggests that even if you directly infiltrate and traumatise the nerve with your needle then it should fully rejuvenate within two months.

You cannot accurately predict the path of the supraorbital nerve; however, as with most complications, the chances of neuropraxia or neuralgia are decreased by understanding the relevant anatomy of your treatment area. The chances of it occurring again in the same patient will be decreased by keeping accurate notes after each treatment and carefully documenting the locations of your injection sites.

## PTOSIS

Ptosis (eyelid droop) can occur after treating the orbicularis oculi muscles or glabellar complex due to botulinum toxin migrating or being directly inoculated into the levator palpebrae superioris or superior tarsal muscles. Patients often present with ptosis on day one or two post-procedure. Ptosis is more likely to occur should you not respect the advised margin of the superior orbital rim or by treating the frontalis or orbicularis oculi muscles lateral to the mid-pupillary line. The risk of ptosis can be further decreased by ensuring that your needle points away from the orbit *at all times* when injecting.

If a patient represents with ptosis after treatment, then perform a thorough ophthalmic assessment and review your case notes. Carefully document the degree of ptosis and correlate this with your injection sites and techniques as well as review the pre- and post-procedure photographs to ensure that the ptosis was not present pre-treatment. Botulinum toxin–induced ptosis should last for between three to four months after treatment. Apologise to your patient and admit that this is likely due to the botulinum toxin treatment to maintain your duty of candour.

There is some evidence that apraclonidine 0.5% eye drops may be beneficial in reducing the severity and length of ptosis due to botulinum toxin treatment. Apraclonidine is an alpha-adrenergic receptor antagonist frequently used in the treatment of glaucoma. It is inadvisable for you to start this treatment in the community without a prior specialist ophthalmology review. Should you cause a ptosis in your patient then best practice would dictate for you to arrange for an urgent ophthalmology assessment for further management. As with all complications, write a letter to the accepting doctor outlining the initial treatment and steps you have taken to rectify this complication.

## HEADACHE

Headache is a relatively common side effect from botulinum toxin treatment and occurs in as many as one in 100 patients treated. Despite being so common, the pathophysiology of a post-procedure headache is relatively poorly understood. Hypotheses into this include increased contraction of facial muscles trying to combat the paralysis induced by botulinum toxin, impurities in the drug itself and direct trauma to the periosteum of the frontal bone or muscle groups treated.

Fortunately, headaches after botulinum toxin treatment are usually rather short-lived and self-limiting. Recommend your patient take a simple over-the-counter analgesic, such as paracetamol for the next few days, until the pain subsides. As headaches are a rather non-specific symptom, advise your patients that should the nature of their headache change, or should they develop neurological symptoms to seek an urgent medical opinion as the botulinum toxin therapy may be a confounder to another pathological process. If a patient suffers a headache after botulinum toxin administration, then they are more likely to suffer headaches from further treatment.

Counsel them to this end before any subsequent treatments to ensure that they are able to give proper informed consent.

## NEW WRINKLE FORMATION

The appearance of new dynamic wrinkles after botulinum toxin are not a complication *per se*; however, they are important potential side effects of treatment which you should discuss with your patients beforehand. Should your treatment be successful, then your patient will have paralysis of the regions treated, yet the surrounding muscles will be as mobile as ever. As the amount of overlying skin remains constant, wrinkling of the area surrounding treatment in a concertina effect is a relatively common occurrence. These new wrinkles are most likely to form in the superior margins of the frontalis and in the region of the temporalis muscles.

Should a patient notice new wrinkles, then take the time to carefully examine them at their review two weeks after treatment. Inform your patient that treatment of these new areas will likely eliminate the wrinkles; however, there will be an increased risk of eyebrow droop or ptosis, especially should the wrinkles be in the temporalis region. Should your patient be keen for a "frozen" appearance, then this may be an acceptable approach, but if they wish to retain some movement, then many patients find it an acceptable consequence of treatment.

The treatment of new wrinkles is straightforward; simply administer half of the advised dose for that region directly into the site of the new wrinkles. This should successfully paralyse the area responsible for new wrinkles, smoothing out the entire treatment area. Ensure you consent your patients for eyebrow droop, ptosis and further new wrinkle formation before undertaking this corrective procedure as these additional injections confer a further risk of complications.

# 11 Introduction to dermal fillers

Dermal fillers are widely used in cosmesis and allow for both augmentation and restoration of lost volume. There are a wide variety of different types of dermal fillers available for purchase, and it is imperative you choose the correct filler for the task at hand. Failure to identify and utilise the correct filler for the required treatment can have disastrous consequences for your patients. In this chapter, we discuss some of the common subtypes of dermal fillers, their advised functions and how the body responds to dermal filler treatments.

Choosing the correct filler for your planned procedure is as important as understanding the correct technique and relevant anatomy to allow you to introduce it safely. It is not only cosmesis which is affected by improper filler choice, but there are also increased risks of complications such as avascular necrosis and delayed onset nodules.

## HYALURONIC ACID

Hyaluronic acid (HA) fillers are the most widely used dermal fillers in Europe and the United States, and their primary mechanism of action is to either replace HA (and therefore volume) lost during the ageing process, or to add more volume to the soft tissues of the face for cosmetic augmentation. HA is a naturally occurring, anionic, non-sulfated glycosaminoglycan consisting of repeat disaccharide units of glucuronic acid and N-acetylglucosamine which can frequently be found within epithelial, neural and epithelial tissues. In humans, up to 50% of our total body HA is located within the skin.

HA is unique amongst glycosaminoglycans as it is produced by bound proteins on the inside of the plasma membrane of *fasciacyte cells*, whereas most other glycosaminoglycans are produced by the Golgi apparatus. The enzymes which synthesise hyaluronic acid are known as HA synthases, and in humans, there are three subtypes: HAS 1, HAS 2 and HAS 3. Each of these enzymatic subtypes will create hyaluronic acid polymers of different chain lengths.

Once formed, hyaluronic acid is secreted through pores in the plasma membrane into the extracellular matrix, where it offers a variety of functions such as hydration, joint lubrication, adding volume, and construction of the extracellular matrix itself. HA also plays a key role in wound healing by helping to activate immune cells and regulate fibroblast and epithelial cell responses to a soft-tissue injury. The length of hyaluronic acid molecules is deterministic in its role in the inflammatory response, with larger molecules (in excess of 1,000 kDa) acting as both an antiangiogenic and immunosuppressive agent, yet smaller molecules are potent inducers of both

DOI: 10.1201/9781003198840-11

inflammation and angiogenesis. Therefore HA dermal fillers with smaller molecules may render a patient more prone to post-procedural swelling than those with larger chain lengths.

The location of hyaluronic acid within the skin differs depending on the individual dermal and epidermal layers. It is predominantly extracellular in the stratum spinosum and granulosum and mainly intracellular in the dermis. Intracellular HA within the dermis and extracellular hyaluronic acid within the deep epidermis draws in water to keep these cells hydrated. This is achieved by having dermal HA concentrations changing in continuum with surrounding lymphatic and vascular structures, allowing for regulation of osmotic pressure and ion flow to maintain a tissue hydration.

As it is a naturally occurring substance, the human body has various methods of degrading and recycling the constituents of HA to ensure the correct concentration is present both within cells and the extracellular matrix. It is estimated that each day, our body degrades and synthesises approximately 30% of its overall volume within the body. The principal group of enzymes for breaking down hyaluronic acid are *hyaluronidases*, which break down HA into oligosaccharides and very low molecular-weight HA. Along with controlled enzymatic degradation, HA is also broken down in an uncontrolled manner by ultraviolet (UV) light, oxidative stress, extremes of temperature and pH changes. These uncontrolled methods of degradation are important to be aware of as both a natural aspect of the ageing process as well as when counselling your patients for post-procedure care after dermal filler treatment.

Both the length of HA chains and overall volume produced decrease as we age. The effect of this change is that our skin loses one of its primary mechanisms of remaining hydrated which results in dehydration, atrophy and decreased elasticity of our epidermal and dermal layers. Research suggests that one of the key mediators in this response is UV light, with sun-exposed areas in the same patient having a lower concentration of HA than sun-covered areas. It is hypothesised therefore that the aggregative effect of solar damage to the skin contributes significantly to the loss of HA in older people.

## HA DERMAL FILLERS

HA within dermal fillers has a different molecular make-up to those encountered in nature, as naturally occurring HA has poor biomechanical properties and a short half-life. These flaws mean that should we administer naturally occurring hyaluronic acid it would add very little volume and not last very long *in vivo*. Nearly all hyaluronic acid fillers on the market today are produced by fermentation of bacteria such as *Streptococcus equii*. The pharmacology of dermal fillers is dependent on a multitude of factors determined by the production processes of each manufacturer, including particle size, cross-linking agent used, the amount of free HA present and rheological properties. Each of these factors individually influences the characteristics of each filler, such as the clinical indication, ease of injection, volume created and side effects. It is worth noting that previously fillers have been determined as mono or biphasic, depending on the homogeneity of HA and the degree of cross-linking. Monophasic dermal fillers are composed of *homogeneous* high or low molecular-weight HA particles, whereas biphasic dermal fillers contain cross-linked HA particles within non-cross-linked HA vehicles and thus are a *heterogeneous* solution. It is worth noting, however, that recent research suggests that this is a failure in nomenclature and these terms should be avoided.

Larger hyaluronic acid particles are more hydrophilic than smaller ones, which means that fillers with larger particles will cause more localised oedema post-treatment and respond more strongly to a patient's hydration status in the long run. Patients treated with larger particle fillers may notice that the region augmented appears plumper when they have drunk a lot of water. Increased cross-linking and concentration of hyaluronic acid particles result in dermal fillers which are both more viscous and have more elastic properties. Cross-linking also determines the cohesivity of dermal fillers and the level of attraction between HA polymers. In essence, cohesivity is the internal adhesive properties holding a HA gel together. Cohesivity is a key factor in the ability for fillers to resist vertical stress, with highly cohesive fillers maintaining their position far better than those which are less cohesive. As cohesion relates to adhesion, it is also worth noting that low cohesion fillers are less likely to remain in their correct tissue plane and are more likely to inadvertently migrate into undesired locations with subsequent loss of cosmetic effect. For example, a more cohesive filler is less likely to migrate above the top of the vermilion border when augmenting the lips and cause an unsightly "shelf" of skin superior to the injection site.

## CONCEPTS OF RHEOLOGY

Rheology is the study of the flow of matter and can be applied to *soft solids* such as a dermal filler and allows for characterisation and assessment of *viscoelasticity*. There are four main parameters to understand when assessing viscoelastic properties:

- $G*$ is the overall viscoelastic property or hardness.
- $G'$ is the measurement of elastic properties.
- $G''$ is the measurement of viscosity.
- Tan $\delta$ is the ratio between viscous and elastic properties.

In essence, a more viscous filler will be firmer and offer more structural support to allow for sculpting or addition of volume to deeper tissues such as the cheeks, nose and chin, whereas more elastic fillers will frequently offer less volume but greater movement and are a sensible choice for fine lines and highly mobile areas. The factors which are most commonly considered are the $G'$, $G''$ and $G'$, $G''$ when choosing where to introduce the filler. The true rheology of a dermal filler is always a trade-off, as should a filler be too viscous and inelastic, then it will be almost impossible to introduce it to tissues with a small needle, whereas elastic and low-cohesivity fillers may not be able to withstand the compressive and shear forces subjected on them during facial movement and will offer no real cosmetic benefit.

Understanding the rheology of the fillers you choose will aid your decision as to which filler is correct for a particular anatomical site. When considering the viscous properties of your filler, you must consider the shear stresses they will be subjected to. Once you have inserted a filler, it will be continuously subjected to forces such as *lateral shear* and *intrinsic* and *extrinsic* compression and stretching. Examples of these are detailed in Table 11.1.

---

**TABLE 11.1**
**Examples of Forces Exerted on Dermal Fillers**

| Force | Example |
|---|---|
| Intrinsic compression | Frowning, pouting |
| Extrinsic compression | Resting face on a surface, kissing |
| Intrinsic lateral shear | Smiling, talking |
| Extrinsic lateral shear | Wiping make-up off face, shaving |

---

It is unlikely that you will choose fillers solely for their elastic modulus and many manufacturers kindly detail the advised anatomical depth and site for injection in their product specification, yet even a brief appreciation of how these influence filler choices are beneficial in understanding *why* a certain filler is a sensible choice (Table 11.2).

---

**TABLE 11.2**
**Physical Properties of Dermal Fillers in Relation to Their Suggested Anatomical Plane**

| Filler Depth | Physical Properties |
|---|---|
| Fine lines | Low cohesivity and medium/low G* and G'. The overall effect will be smooth, subtle increased volume with a low risk of visible edges or lumps. |
| Midface | G' able to sustain shearing and medium/high compression forces. These fillers will be able to add volume and sculpt the face without succumbing to the strong tension and forces required to move the lips and cheeks. |
| Lower face | Moderate/low cohesivity and moderate G'. A combination of these factors will allow fillers to restore volume in areas such as marionette lines but to remain elastic enough for facial movements to be unimpeded and visible lumps not be demonstrated |
| Nose and chin | High cohesivity and high G' to allow fillers to retain their shape whilst resisting the high compressive and shear forces of the soft tissues overlying the nose and chin. High cohesivity and high G' fillers are less likely to migrate and will result in a vertical projection for a longer time to enable sufficient sculpting of these areas |

---

HYALURONIC ACID DERMAL FILLERS: PHYSIOLOGY

As dermal fillers are a foreign body and that you are traumatising tissues whilst introducing them, it is unsurprising that there is associated localised oedema after treatment. You can counsel your patients that the oedema is likely to be most pronounced the morning after treatment and this will resolve over the next two to

14 days to allow them to avoid any undue concern once the swelling has arisen. Post-procedural swelling is at its greatest the morning after treatment due to both the time taken for an established inflammatory response to occur, as well as the gravitational effects on interstitial fluid whilst sleeping lying flat. The chances of swelling can be reduced by advising your patients to sleep upright the night of your treatment; however, many patients find this uncomfortable and will frequently risk increased swelling for a more comfortable night's sleep.

The duration of hyaluronic acid fillers is highly variable and is dependent on

- lifestyle factors such as smoking and avoiding excessive sunlight,
- patient-specific factors such as the speed at which they naturally metabolise hyaluronic acid and
- practitioner factors, such as injection technique, rheology and the composition of chosen filler.

In the majority of cases, patients can expect results from HA filler augmentation to last between six to 12 months; however, it is prudent to counsel them that the filler will be permanently metabolised by their body and subsequently will decrease in volume by a minuscule amount on a daily basis. The life span of dermal fillers is decreased by smoking and excessive sunlight, being placed in a highly mobile area (such as the lips) and by poor injection technique, namely injecting the dermal filler deep to the dermis itself.

## CALCIUM HYDROXYAPATITE DERMAL FILLERS

Calcium hydroxyapatite (CaHa) makes up the mineral component of bones and teeth, making them both hard and strong. Approximately half of the volume of the bony skeleton is composed of CaHa crystals deposited on collagen matrices.

In the world of cosmetics, CaHa fillers are comprised of uniform CaHa microspheres with a diameter of 25 µm to 45 µm suspended in a sodium carboxymethylcellulose gel, with a usual ratio of 30% CaHa to 70% sodium carboxymethylcellulose. The carboxymethylcellulose gel is necessary for the CaHa microspheres to be delivered to the desired tissue plane via injection. At the time of writing, CaHa dermal fillers have a Food and Drug Administration licence to treat moderate to severe facial wrinkles and lost volume, such as the nasolabial folds or to treat the cosmetic consequences of HIV lipodystrophy.

Due to its molecular mimicry of the mineral part of bone, CaHa metabolism is strikingly similar to that of bony fragments after a fracture. Between 8 to 12 weeks after treatment, the carboxylmethylcellulose gel is absorbed and replaced by newly synthesised collagen. CaHa also functions by acting as a scaffold onto which new tissues can be grown, causing localised fibroblast activation within the dermal layer to which they are injected. There has been no evidence as of yet to suggest that CaHa microspheres enter bone cortices or cause any consequent calcification. Research suggests that there is excellent immunocompatibility and tolerance to treatment with CaHa fillers, with a minimal inflammatory response and no foreign body response or systemic toxicity demonstrated.

## POLY-L-LACTIC ACID DERMAL FILLERS

The mechanism of action of poly-L-lactic acid varies significantly compared to the other common dermal filler subtypes. It is believed to function by stimulating dermal fibroblasts to undergo neocollagenesis and therefore can be considered a dermal *stimulator* as opposed to a dermal *filler*. As it relies of neocollagenesis to restore lost volume, it is important to counsel your patients that they may not see results for up to eight weeks after treatment and that many patients require multiple treatments – typically three treatments every three weeks – to stimulate sufficient collagen regrowth to have the desired effect.

Poly-L-lactic acid fillers are usually reconstituted with 5 mL of sterile water and left to stand for a minimum of two hours to ensure the molecules are adequately rehydrated. Once reconstituted, the solution should be agitated (such as swirling the vial in your hand) before administration. These fillers are usually introduced to the subdermal layer in a cross-hatch pattern to allow for adequate neocollagenesis to occur. Typical patients treated with poly-L-lactic acid are those with mild-moderate wrinkles.

One of the biggest risks for complications if treated with poly-L-lactic acid is the formation of delayed-onset nodules. These nodules are frequently palpable yet not perceivable with the naked eye. There has been some evidence to suggest that the formation of nodules can be decreased by using a larger volume of water for dilution and with vigorous post-treatment massage. The area at greatest risk of nodule formation is the hands, with as many as one in 10 patients reporting some nodularity after treatment with this product.

## POLYMETHYLMETHACRYLATE DERMAL FILLERS

These fillers are commonly composed of polymethylmethacrylate (PMMA) microspheres within either a bovine collagen or a methylcellulose gel. They are administered into the deep dermis and frequently used to permanently treat nasolabial folds, marionette lines and glabellar creases. Similar to poly-L-lactic acid fillers, the gel is metabolised by the soft tissues of the body in a few weeks to months after delivery, leaving the residual microparticles in situ. These microparticles are believed to then trigger a localised inflammatory response and become surrounded by a fibrous capsule deposited by macrophages and fibroblasts. As part of this process, neocollagenesis ensues with newly synthesised collagen molecules being deposited on these fibrous capsules with subsequent volumising effects.

As many PMMA fillers are partially comprised of a bovine collagen gel, you must consent your patients to this before treatment as they may have religious or ethical objections to treatment. It is also imperative that you undertake an allergy skin test four weeks before treatment with PMMA fillers to ensure your patient does not have an allergic reaction to these products.

Table 11.3 shows some of the more commonly utilised dermal fillers within the United Kingdom, outlining their primary constituents and the areas which they are commonly used to treat.

**TABLE 11.3**
**Examples of Common Dermal Fillers**

| Product Name | Constituent | Manufacturer | Frequently treated areas |
|---|---|---|---|
| Belotero Soft | Hyaluronic acid | Merz | Superficial wrinkles |
| Belotero Basic | Hyaluronic acid | Merz | Moderate/deep wrinkles<br>Lip augmentation |
| Belotero Intense | Hyaluronic acid | Merz | Deep wrinkles<br>Lip augmentation |
| Juvedérm Ultra 2 | Hyaluronic acid | Allergan | Superficial wrinkles |
| Juvedérm Ultra 3 | Hyaluronic acid | Allergan | Moderate/deep wrinkles<br>Lips |
| Juvedérm Ultra 4 | Hyaluronic acid | Allergan | Deep depressions<br>Lip augmentation<br>Cheekbone augmentation |
| Juvedérm Ultra Smile | Hyaluronic acid | Allergan | Lip augmentation<br>Perioral lines |
| Juvedérm Voluma | Hyaluronic acid | Allergan | Contouring cheeks/jawline/chin |
| Restylane | Hyaluronic acid | Galderma | Moderate facial wrinkles<br>Including nasolabial folds and marionette lines |
| Restylane Perlane | Hyaluronic acid | Galderma | Deep wrinkles<br>Cheek volumisation |
| Restylane Lip Volume | Hyaluronic acid | Galderma | Lip Augmentation |
| Restylane SubQ | Hyaluronic acid | Galderma | Hydration of neck/acne scars/décolletage/hands |
| Teosyal Global Action | Hyaluronic acid | Teoxane | Moderate wrinkles |
| Teosyal Kiss | Hyaluronic acid | Teoxane | Lip augmentation |
| Teosyal Deep Lines | Hyaluronic acid | Teoxane | Deep wrinkles |
| Teosyal Ultra Deep | Hyaluronic acid | Teoxane | Cheekbone/chin augmentation |
| Sculptra | Poly-L-lactic acid | Dermik aesthetic | Wrinkles/facial volume los |
| Radiesse | Calcium hydroxyapatite | Merz | Moderate/severe facial wrinkles |
| Artecoll | Rofil medical | Polymethylmethacrylate | Deep wrinkles |

# 12 Dermal fillers
## *Practical skills*

## PREPARATION

Arguably the most important part of performing any treatment is preparing your patient properly, and failure to do so will likely not only decrease the chances of a satisfactory cosmetic outcome but may also put your patient at undue risk.

Before your patient has even entered your consultation room, ensure that you have your treatment couch in an area of adequate lighting with enough space to manoeuvre. Consider whether you wish to be standing or sitting whilst administering dermal fillers and have the couch at a height from which you can comfortably reach the areas which you are aiming to treat. Finally, take the time to check you have all the necessary equipment you need and that it is within easy reach from your treatment position in a manner in which you can maintain sterility.

Once you are satisfied with the preceding, and you and your patient have reached a shared decision on treatment, invite them to the treatment couch. It is often advisable to perform dermal filler augmentation (and botulinum toxin administration) with the patient lying flat. This affords you greater control over their soft tissues, makes the relevant anatomy more predictable, and decreases the chances of your patient having a vasovagal syncope. Some patients will not be able to tolerate lying flat. Should this be the case, then try to position as close to horizontal as they find comfortable. Take your before photos once they are positioned appropriately, ensuring to take at least one image from directly in front of the patient and one of each size. These photographs will be the core of any further treatment plans and are a necessary part of your patient's medical documentation and must be retained within your patient's notes.

After taking the necessary photographs, put on some gloves and clean the treatment area with an alcohol swab (or similar) as outlined in Chapter 9. Once the area has air-dried, apply liberal amounts of topical anaesthetic such as 5% lidocaine cream. Topical anaesthesia will not completely numb the area, yet it will make the treatment more tolerable until the local anaesthetic in your dermal filler of choice has taken effect. Topical lidocaine usually takes five minutes or so to take effect, so use this time to double-check you have all the necessary equipment and sundries to undertake treatment as well as answer any last-minute questions your patient may have. Once you are satisfied, should your patient still give consent, then re-sterilise the area and proceed.

## NASOLABIAL FOLDS

Nasolabial folds are skin creases from the nasal alar which extend inferolaterally adjacent to the corners of the mouth. They become more prominent as we age due to the intrinsic loss of volume and elasticity within the cheeks and a lifetime of

DOI: 10.1201/9781003198840-12

repeated facial movements. As these creases become more apparent as patients get older, many people seek dermal filler augmentation to smoothen these lines and thus make them less prominent.

The treatment of nasolabial folds is usually in the form of a retrograde linear injection, with the volume administered dependent on the depth of the folds themselves. In most cases, nasolabial folds can be treated with an intermediate viscosity filler. Prepare your treatment by accurately measuring the length of the nasolabial fold in terms of needle lengths by resting your needle along its length and measuring in a stepwise manner from the proximal aspect to the distal end of the fold. Try to imagine that you will be doing a series of contiguous injections in order to make a stable and even line of filler (Figure 12.1). Always be liberal with the use of topical local anaesthetic in the region of injection as it is a notoriously painful place to treat.

Take special care when sterilising and preparing the area for augmentation with dermal fillers as the nasolabial folds make up the lateral borders of the "triangle of

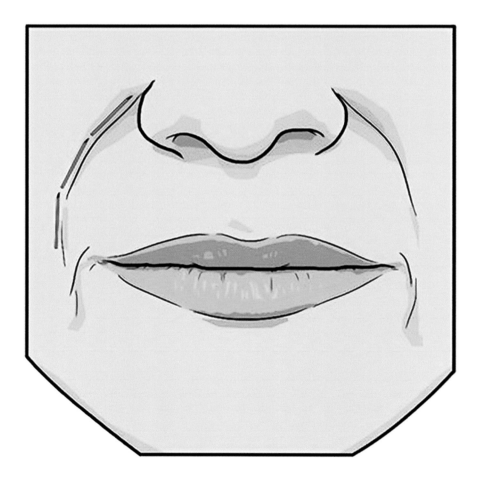

**FIGURE 12.1**  Approximation of needle lengths for the treatment of nasolabial folds.

danger" of the face. Should filler enter a vein in this region, or should you inadvertently cause an infection, there is a chance that retrograde infection or filler embolus could result in cavernous sinus thrombosis, meningitis or a cerebral abscess. Due to these risks, ensure that you not only maintain the aseptic non-touch technique but also always draw back on the syringe before injecting. Should you see a "flashback" of blood on aspiration then re-site the needle and try again to prevent accidental injection of filler within a blood vessel.

Once you are happy with your proposed needle placement, pull the skin tight with your thumb and index finger. This will distort the local anatomy so take care to check that you are indeed injecting in the correct site to prevent undesirable cosmesis. Your injections will be slightly deeper than when treating the lips, and correct needle depth is accepted as being able to see the *outline* of the needle without seeing its grey colour.

When injecting you will notice that the pressure required to expel your filler is greater than when treating the lips due to denser connective tissue of the cheeks. Slowly administer the filler whilst simultaneously withdrawing your needle as the same speed as the filler is injected. Never inject whilst the needle is stationary as this increases the chances of both complications and a poor cosmetic outcome due to a bolus of filler. Stop injecting just before you remove your needle from the skin, as continuing to inject until the needle is fully withdrawn can result in accidental epidermal deposition of dermal filler which may result in soft-tissue nodule formation. Special care needs to be taken when injecting the superior portion of the fold as a bolus in this region can result in an undesirable filler lump, the Tyndall effect or in severe cases avascular necrosis.

Best practice dictates that you treat one nasolabial fold as a series of linear retrograde injections before doing the second. Try not to focus too much on the *volume* of filler administered but more so bilateral symmetry. Patients often have one fold which is deeper than the other, so should you try to put an equal amount of filler in each side, you may result in asymmetrical nasolabial folds once you have finished.

You may find that augmentation with a middle-thickness filler is insufficient in patients with deeper nasolabial folds. In these circumstances, you may wish to insert a deeper and thicker filler inferior to the middle thickness filler of your choosing. This adds volume to the deep dermis or subcutaneous layer to make deeper lines less noticeable and can be done before or after your primary treatment.

Once you have treated the nasolabial folds, run your thumb down the region treated in a craniocaudal direction to smooth the filler and decrease the chance of any lumps forming.

## MARIONETTE LINES

Marionette lines are vertical lines extending inferiorly from the corner of the mouth, with their name deriving from the characteristic appearance of the mouths of string puppets. These lines are due to age-related volume loss and movement of the mouth. Many patients state that their marionette lines give them a "sad" appearance due to the volume loss causing a slight down-turning of the corners of the mouth.

There are three methods of treating marionette lines depending on the degree of volume loss and level of support you wish to create. These are *linear retrograde injections*, *fanning* and *cross-hatching*. Most practitioners find that an intermediate viscosity filler is sufficient for decreasing the visibility of these lines.

### LINEAR RETROGRADE TECHNIQUE

Linear retrograde injections are best utilised in treating more superficial skin creases. In most instances, one needle length will be sufficient to treat the entirety of the line. Pull the skin tight and insert your needle within the dermis deep to the line itself, with the correct depth being demonstrated as being able to see the outline of your needle without being able to see the grey colour. Inject slowly in a linear retrograde manner, taking care not to bolus the proximal part of the line and to not have filler extrude from your puncture site. Bear in mind that the labial artery and vein enter at the corner of the mouth, so ensure that you have not entered it by pulling back your syringe before injecting. Overfilling at this site can easily cause vascular occlusion with devastating consequences. See Figure 12.2.

Should you need to both treat the line *and* restore volume inferior to the corners of the mouth due to a "sad" appearance, then you may wish to consider cross-hatching or fanning as the method of introducing filler. Both techniques allow for a relatively high concentration of filler to be placed within tissues without needing to administer a bolus which may cause an undesirable lump. Adding volume inferolaterally to the angles of the mouth will cause them to angle upwards slightly and turn a sad appearing mouth into a happier looking one.

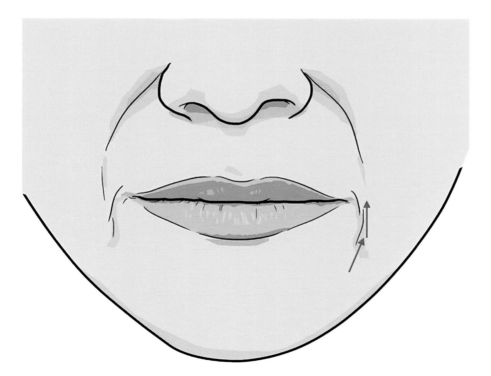

**FIGURE 12.2**   Approximate needle positioning for retrograde linear injections for the treatment of marionette lines.

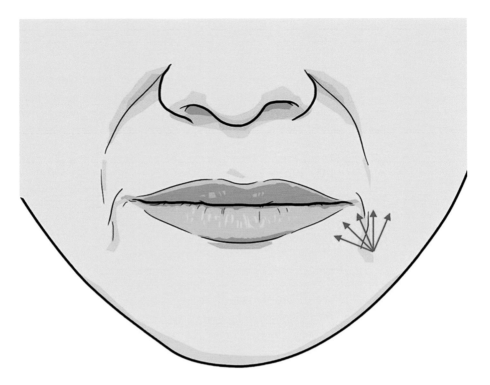

**FIGURE 12.3** The "fanning" technique for treatment of marionette lines.

### FANNING

Fanning is a useful technique to improve volume and apply a buttress of filler to support an area of volume loss (Figure 12.3). Plan your procedure by lining up your needle along the length of the line with the tip pointing cranially then angle your needle at 30° either side of this to get your eye in. Pull the skin taut and insert your needle into the dermis 45° medial to the crease itself and perform a linear retrograde injection. Do not remove your needle from the skin once you have reached the end, and instead reinsert it with a slight lateral angulation and repeat until you have reached 45° lateral to the line itself. The result of this technique is that you are administering multiple retrograde linear injections from one puncture site, decreasing pain and discomfort to the patient whilst increasing volume.

### CROSS-HATCHING

Cross-hatching has a similar volumising effect to fanning and is arguably more stable at the expense of being more traumatic to the soft tissues of your patient (Figure 12.4). This procedure will involve four or nine injections in a grid, either two by two or three by three. Your injection sites will be inferolateral to the corner of the mouth, deep to the marionette line and area of volume loss. Once you have sterilised

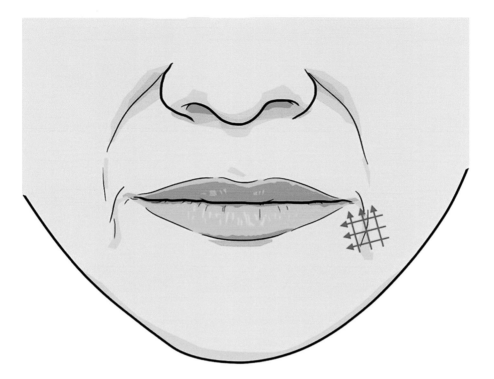

**FIGURE 12.4** The "cross-hatching" technique for treatment of marionette lines.

the skin and pulled it tight, insert your needle its entire length with the line. You should aim for the centre of the marionette line to be halfway down the shaft of your needle. Perform two or three parallel linear retrograde injections and then repeat the process over the same area at 90° to your primary injection. This will create a cross-hatch of filler to add both volume and support to this area. Ensure you smooth down the region with your thumb afterwards to ensure that there are no lumps present.

## LIP AUGMENTATION

Lip augmentation is one of the most popular treatment areas with dermal fillers, especially in younger females. When augmenting the lips you need to insert your needle at a relatively acute angle to the skin (somewhere in the region of 20°) in order to infiltrate the superficial dermis. Superficial dermal infiltration will allow you to add volume and shape to lips, yet it comes with increased risk of causing a lumpy texture due to a relative paucity of overlying soft tissue. See Figure 12.5.

You will, as your practice continues, develop your own style of lip augmentation based on your understanding of how patients respond to lip filler as well as in creating your patient's desired cosmetic outcome. This chapter gives you a brief overview of techniques with which you can augment lips effectively and safely.

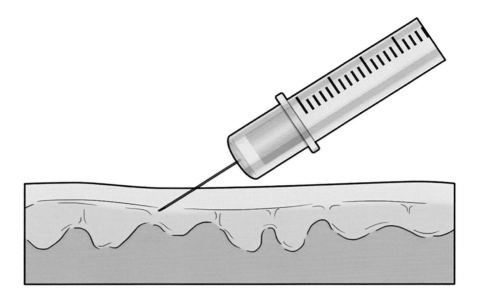

**FIGURE 12.5**    Correct needle angulation for lip augmentation.

Before you start augmenting a patient's lips, take the time to explore with them what look they are after and what they are particularly interested in changing. Lip augmentation is not simply about making lips *bigger*, but you can also correct asymmetry or change the shape of the lips themselves.

It is imperative that you assess the lips of your patient in detail before starting any treatment, not only checking for contraindications but also to see if you can deliver a realistic outcome. Should a person attend with very thin lips, then you will be unlikely to be able to safely create large lips after a solitary treatment session. If you are overambitious with the amount of filler you administer then you can overfill an area, distort the patient's anatomy, decrease the acuity of or have filler migrate superiorly to the vermilion border, making their lips appear smaller than before you started.

Initially it is useful to lay down a foundation of filler to act as a support for further augmentation. In the vast majority of patients, it is worthwhile injecting filler in the shape of an "M" around the lateral and medial aspects of the Cupid's bow as a series of linear retrograde injections. It is often advisable to begin by treating the top lip, so for your first injection start by inserting your needle into the dermal layer just below the vermilion border approximately one needle length from the peak of the Cupid's bow. Advance your needle from a lateral approach and to the tip of the Cupid's bow on that side before performing your first linear retrograde injection. See Figure 12.6.

Once you have done this, do the same on the other side and check for symmetry. To augment the middle of the Cupid's bow, follow the same principles but start with your needle within the lowermost point of the middle of the top lip with the tip yet

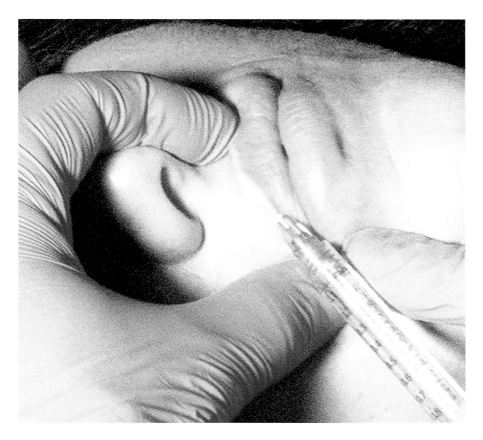

**FIGURE 12.6** Correct needle depth for lip augmentation.

again sited within the apex of the bow itself on that side. Always perform these injections via a linear retrograde technique, as boluses within the lip can not only cause unsightly lumps but also confer an increased risk of vascular occlusion and subsequent avascular necrosis.

Once you have augmented the Cupid's bow, you may wish to perform one further linear retrograde injection on either side of the top lip running horizontally approximately halfway from the tip of the Cupid's bow to the wet-dry border of the lip. For these injections, introduce your needle at the lateral aspect of the lip, yet again just below the vermilion border, and insert it to the hilt (should there be space to do so). This step will allow you to add further volume to the top lip with relative ease. Always avoid introducing your needle or injecting filler at the corner of the mouth, as this is where the labial arteries and veins enter the lips; therefore, traumatising or introducing filler within this region has an unacceptably high change of causing damage to these vessels and avascular necrosis secondary to either a localised haematoma or the filler itself.

After you have placed a foundation in the top lip, administer four injections to the bottom lip: two centrally and one to each side of this (Figure 12.7). Yet again inject lateromedially on the sides, and for the middle inject one right to left and the other left to right to decrease the chance of lateral asymmetry. Inject one middle injection inferiorly and one superiorly to ensure that you increase volume without creating a *trout pout*.

Once you have laid down your foundation, give your patient the chance to objectively critique your work so far. Give them a hand-held mirror and ask them to take the time to have a detailed look at the augmentation you have performed. Reassure them that you won't be offended, nor are you seeking compliments, yet an honest answer will allow you to continue with the procedure and makes your patient having their desired outcome far more likely. This foundation will be the base of the rest of your augmentation for this patient, so in particular, make sure they are happy with the overall shape you have created. Ask them to specifically comment on any asymmetry or bowing of the lips to allow you to rectify it immediately. At this step, you should also take the time to explore how they would like to proceed with treatment, for example changing the shape of the lips or further increasing volume before resuming augmentation.

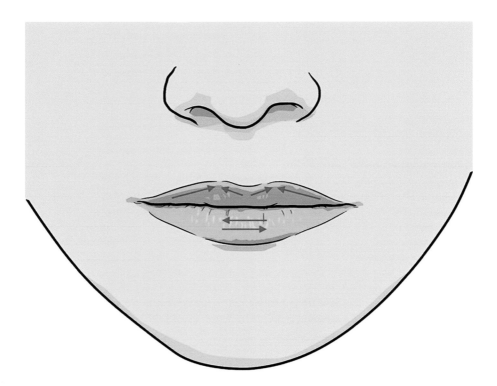

**FIGURE 12.7**    Standard injection technique for lip augmentation.

It is worthwhile to then discuss further options with your patient. Most patients will have an idea of what look they are after, and they will require your expertise in not only delivering the desired cosmesis but also to be able to offer the impartial advice on whether their desired outcome will suit their face.

### WIDENING THE LIPS

Laterally you can fill lips down to a few millimetres from the corner of the mouth to decrease the chances of vascular occlusion. This has an affect of widening the lips as well as creating a "lip curl" which some patients may request. Bear in mind that if your patient has vertically small lips, then filling too laterally runs the risk of making the mouth relatively too wide. This will not confer a desirable overall cosmetic outcome. Widening the lips is usually most advisable in patients with more pronounced features such as a strong nose, high cheekbones, or wide jaw. Commonly if you were to do this on a patient with more delicate features, the mouth would appear unnaturally prominent and detract from their face as a whole. See Figure 12.8.

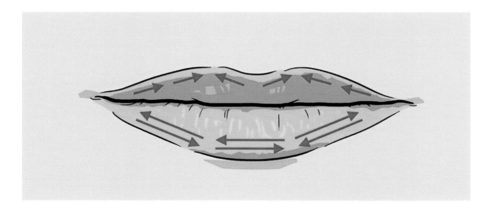

**FIGURE 12.8**    Injection techniques for widening the lips.

### "DOLLY LIPS"

This approach is best utilised in patients with delicate facial features, so as to not make the mouth the focal point and in keeping with their facial structure. When treating such a patient, try to avoid any injections in the lateral third of the mouth on either side. Perform the aforementioned *M* augmentation with reinforcing lateral injections inferior to this. In the bottom lip, introduce four horizontal injections parallel and adjacent to one another. This will create volume without widening the lip and detracting from the patient's natural appearance (Figure 12.9).

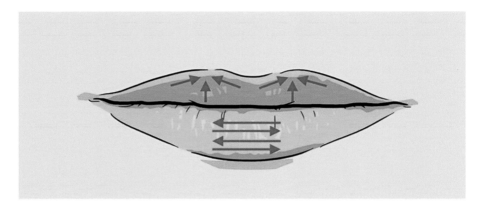

**FIGURE 12.9**    Injection techniques to create "dolly lips".

## Lifting the top lip

Should your patient want a lift in their top lip, then you may wish to place two injections with the needle immediately above the wet–dry border and aiming superiorly. Yet again perform a retrograde linear injection with the initial injection in the top of the Cupid's bow. This should lift the entire top lip without running the risk of creating a sausage-like appearance. To support these injections, consider two further injections in the midline such as you would when adding volume to the bottom lip. This should create a lift in the top lip if performed correctly (Figure 12.10).

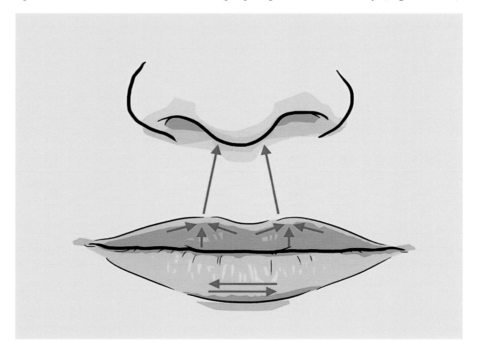

**FIGURE 12.10**    Injection techniques to lift the top lip.

This technique (along with the *M* foundation discussed earlier) is especially useful for patients who have an ill-defined top lip. In such patients, you may also want to consider infiltrating the prominences of the philtrum to lift the top lip and create a more defined Cupid's bow. If you wish to infiltrate the philtrum, insert your needle inferiorly to its anterior fold where it joins the lip through the apex of the Cupid's bow on the lip itself. Introduce your needle its entire length and perform a retrograde linear injection. The correct depth of this procedure is the same as with the nasolabial folds; you should be able to see the outline *but not the grey colour* of the needle.

## Thin lips

You may find it difficult to augment a patient with thin lips when starting out on your practice. If a patient with thin lips presents to you wanting noticeably larger lips then a fair degree of forward planning is required to create their desired cosmetic effects. Counsel these patients that you may not be able to deliver their desired outcome, and that if you wish to it will likely take a series of injections over several months.

When treating a thinner-lipped individual it is best to start with 0.5 mL of a middle-thickness filler. Take the time to create an M-shaped foundation for the Cupid's bow with associated vertical and horizontal midline injections. Take the time to also administer the standard four lower lip injections in these patients and then stop. Do not be disheartened if you do not have a significant cosmetic effect after this treatment; however, it is essential to do this to prepare for your next therapy.

Arrange to meet your patient in 8–12 weeks after this treatment. This should allow for the tissues of the lips to have accommodated the filler whilst preserving the desired shape and vermilion border. When you see them for the second therapy, administer up to a maximum of 1 mL of middle-thickness filler. In these instances it is best to repeat the previous injections you have already administered, as well as consider introducing further lateral injections. This gentle approach will respect the tissues of the lips as well as will allow you to safely create space to insert dermal filler and create volume.

Should your patient still want further augmentation or additional volume, then leave it a minimum of another three months before augmenting their lips once more. It is advisable, should you choose to do so, would be to only administer a maximum of 0.5 mL further hyaluronic acid. Administrating >2 mL in one calendar year greatly increases the chances of infection, lip lumps and distorted tissue planes.

## CHEEK AUGMENTATION

Augmenting the cheeks is a common procedure in both younger patients wanting more defined cheekbones as well as older patients aiming to replace lost volume. Administration of cheek fillers is different in principle to the majority of dermal filler injections as it is performed at a 90° angle to the skin, much like botulinum toxin injections. The needle used is often longer and of a large calibre than used for other soft tissue augmentation to enable the introduction of a viscous filler *just above* the periosteum. Be careful in any patient who has had previous facial trauma or surgery as this will distort the bony anatomy of the maxilla and zygoma and result in aberrant muscular, vascular or neural anatomy. Should you have a patient with a history of craniofacial trauma or surgery it is inadvisable to proceed with treatment unless you are certain you will not inadvertently cause any harm.

The first step in cheek augmentation is to assess your patient to ensure they are suitable for the treatment. Cheek augmentation may not only restore lost volume in the cheeks but also can decrease the visibility of bags under the eyes or periocular wrinkles on smiling. A quick and easy method of assessing for volume loss in the cheeks is to run your index finger from the zygoma to the nasal bone in a sweeping motion. Corrugation of the skin whilst you perform this motion is likely to indicate volume loss in this area. If a patient is seeking cheek fillers without volume loss, then this test may not be overly useful, and it may not be in their best interests to proceed with treatment.

Once you have decided that a patient is suitable for treatment, follow the contour of the skin under the eye in a curve inferolaterally and a second line laterally from the superior nasal alar in a straight line. The point at which these lines bisect should be the location of your first injection. Be very careful once you have chosen your injection site as the point of your lines bisecting is likely to be very close to *if not directly on top* of the inferior orbital notch. Ensure that you are not likely to traumatise or occlude this area by palpating for the notch with your finger. If you believe you are likely to inject over the inferior orbital notch, then it is advisable to move your needle a few millimetres laterally.

When injecting the filler, introduce the needle perpendicular to the skin with the skin anchored by your non-dominant hand. Slowly insert the needle to the level of the periosteum and then retract it by 1–2 mm. At this point, you can stop anchoring the skin temporarily and withdraw the syringe for five seconds whilst keeping the needle in position. It is good practice to count out loud for five seconds to decrease the chance of rushing this step. Aspiration is one of the most important steps in this procedure, as injecting a viscous filler into an artery or vein would be catastrophic. When you are certain you are safe to inject, then deliver your filler as a bolus with a standard dose for this region being 0.2 mL. Once you have finished, withdraw your needle and apply firm pressure to this site for a few seconds to ensure haemostasis. Your second injection site will be immediately lateral to your first, usually one finger's breadth or so away whilst your third and final injection will be slightly superolateral to your second over the zygomatic process. Your medial injection is also advised to be 0.2 mL and the most lateral 0.1 mL. Do not perform a linear retrograde injection whilst augmenting the cheeks as you are unlikely to add volume but instead incur an increased risk of granuloma or filler nodule formation. See Figure 12.11.

Once you have completed one side, follow the same protocol to treat the contralateral side. Assess your post-treatment outcomes looking at your patient face on as well as with them lying flat and you looking from the head end down. Give your patient a chance to analyse your work and offer feedback regarding potential asymmetry. Should the cheeks be asymmetrical, assess for loss of volume by sweeping your finger across the cheek once more. Asymmetry is easily corrected by administering a small volume of filler to the side with less volume.

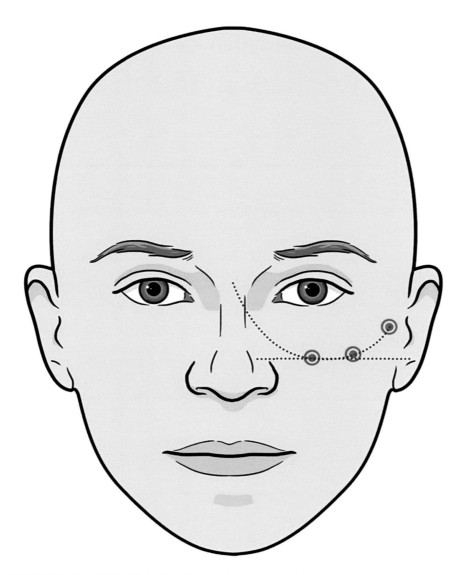

**FIGURE 12.11** Advised injection sites for cheek augmentation.

# 13 Dermal filler complications and management

The complications of dermal filler augmentation are much more widely publicised than those of botulinum toxin therapy. There are multiple reasons why this may be the case; first, at the time of writing, dermal fillers are not a prescription-only medication in the United Kingdom and therefore may be administered by somebody who has undertaken no medical training. Second, due to the variety of fillers available on the market, it is easy for an inexperienced individual to choose the wrong filler to treat a particular area, and finally (and perhaps the most likely reason for their increased prominence) is that dermal filler complications are more likely to result in dramatic outcomes garnering attention on news channels and social media.

Following are various common complications of dermal filler administration in alphabetical order for ease of reference.

## AVASCULAR NECROSIS

Avascular necrosis is the term used to describe cell death secondary to a lack of oxygenated blood. In the context of dermal filler augmentation, there are two main mechanisms in which avascular necrosis can occur: first, it may be caused by direct injection of dermal filler into an artery, and second, it may due to a local pressure effect of the filler itself pressing on an artery from the outside. Regardless of the underlying cause, avascular necrosis can confer devastating long-term sequelae on your patients and therefore mandates swift identification and definitive management.

### PATHOPHYSIOLOGY OF AVASCULAR NECROSIS

When a cell becomes devoid of sufficient oxygen to drive cellular processes, it is deemed *hypoxic*. Oxygen is required to synthesise adenosine triphosphate (ATP) via oxidative phosphorylation, with ATP being used to supply the energy required to drive multiple cellular pathways. When a cell does not have enough oxygen to create ATP and subsequently enough energy to perform metabolic processes, it will die. Hypoxic cell death is a passive process known as *necrosis*. Necrosis is entirely unregulated and not an actively driven or controlled by cellular mediators. When cells cannot continue to perform the necessary functions to survive, the cell membrane will become irregular with the formation of *blebs* and eventually ruptures with release of cellular components into the surrounding tissues. If this were an isolated process, the damage caused would not be overly significant. The body, however, has a protective mechanism which ironically exacerbates the local process of necrosis to prevent systemic damage due to the release of toxins from necrotic cells. Cells which are surrounding an area of necrosis, otherwise known as a penumbra, will commit suicide through a

DOI: 10.1201/9781003198840-13

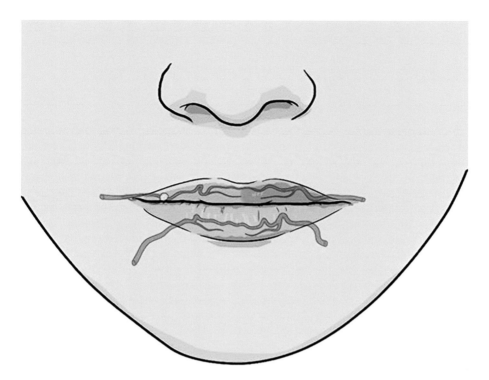

**FIGURE 13.1**   Diagrammatic representation of avascular necrosis secondary to arterial ischaemia.

tightly regulated process called *apoptosis*. This programmed cell death is designed to create a wall around a necrotic cluster of cells to prevent potentially toxic intracellular components from destroying large volumes of surrounding tissue. In apoptosis, cells will flag themselves up to be destroyed, and will break apart in a controlled manner into small vesicles known as apoptotic bodies. These bodies are then phagocytosed, or eaten and digested, by white blood cells called macrophages.

You may be intrigued as to why this level of detail was required as a background into avascular necrosis; however, it is essential to appreciate that the area of potential tissue damage is not solely limited to the area which receives a direct arterial supply from an occluded vessel, but also the penumbra which surrounds it. This understanding is important in counselling patients regarding the prognosis of a hypoxic insult to tissues.

## Danger areas

There are two primary danger zones which are at heightened risk of avascular necrosis:

> *The glabellar region*: approximately half of all reported cases of avascular necrosis occur here. This area is at heightened risk of avascular necrosis due to a lack of collateral arterial supply at this location.

*Nasal tip and alar triangle*: this region is only supplied by one end artery, the angular artery, which has no collateral flow and is easily occluded. To make matters trickier, the angular artery turns tightly within the nasal alar and subsequently is easily compressed by external filler application.

DECREASING THE RISK OF AVASCULAR NECROSIS

The most important factor in decreasing the risk of avascular necrosis is to be aware of the relevant local anatomy of the region which you are treating. If you are unsure of the likely distribution of local blood vessels and surrounding structures, then take the time to refresh your memory by reading Chapter 3 or a dedicated anatomical textbook before undertaking any treatments.

One key consideration is your filler technique. Poor technique increases the chance of almost any complication, and avascular necrosis is no different. Whenever you are treating a patient with dermal fillers, aspirate the syringe before expelling the filler. If, when you aspirate, you get a flashback of blood then you may well be within a vein or artery. Relocate your needle before pulling back again and only inject filler when you are confident you are not within a vascular structure. There is also some evidence that the use of a blunt cannula when injecting may decrease the likelihood of you accidentally invading a vascular structure with your needle; however, should you prefer to use a needle technique then take steps to mitigate the risk by always pulling back on the plunger. It is inadvisable to use an approach in which you are not trained or comfortable, as the risk of complications far less likely to occur in practitioners who are experienced with their chosen technique.

When injecting fillers, ensure that you are injecting at the correct depth for the procedure, and use as small an amount of filler as possible to create the desired cosmetic effect. It is also worth avoiding the use of boluses within areas prone to necrosis to decrease the chances of localised arterial compression. Products which contain adrenaline may make avascular necrosis more likely, as these may cause localised vasoconstriction and consequent tissue hypoxia.

Finally, watch your patient's face when you are treating them, and look out for subtle signs of increased pain. Ask them how the treatment is going, but bear in mind that they may be sufficiently anaesthetised to not feel anything initially. This risk is even greater should a patient have a dental block prior to treatment as it will confer very effective local anaesthesia.

Best practice is to observe the area of treatment for a few minutes once you have finished to check for areas of blanching or discolouration.

MANAGEMENT OF AVASCULAR NECROSIS

Avascular necrosis can be seen in any tissue you infiltrate with dermal fillers; however, as previously discussed, it is most likely to occur in soft tissues overlying the procerus muscle and adjacent to the nasal alar. Some of the initial symptoms are relatively non-specific, and therefore, you must rely on your own clinical judgement in this context. One of the first symptoms a patient may report is acute pain; however, as previously mentioned this may not be noted if the treatment area has been well anaesthetised. The devascularised tissues will begin to exhibit pallor in comparison to surrounding skin almost immediately; however, this does not *definitely* indicate avascular necrosis. Transient pallor after injection may be a normal finding, therefore take the time to observe the tissues for a few seconds to ascertain whether they return to their normal colour or not. If you are unsure as to the nature of any pallor you observe, you can press on the affected area and assess the capillary refill time. This should be less than two seconds; any longer than this may indicate arterial insufficiency and that the patient is indeed at risk of avascular necrosis.

As the remaining oxygen within the tissues is metabolised, all that will remain is a dark-blue discolouration of deoxygenated venous blood. This will eventually turn grey as tissues begin to necrose. Once necrosis has taken hold, a well-demarcated area of tissue necrosis is demonstrated with a hyperaemic border, due to the previously mentioned sequence of necrosis and protective apoptosis. The area of avascular necrosis will have a "punched-out" appearance, as if somebody had neatly cut out a circle of tissue. Finally, several days to weeks after the initial insult, tissues will attempt to repair by a process known as secondary intention, the term used to describe an open wound healing of its own accord.

The preceding process is a brief overview of what you may see in the event of avascular necrosis. It has a high chance of affected tissues becoming scarred or infected, as well as very undesirable cosmesis for your patient. The cascade of necrosis and apoptosis is not preventable once tissues have started to undergo the process, therefore it is important to notice early signs (such as delayed capillary refill, blanching of the skin, and an eventual blueish hue) and treat the patient accurately and effectively. There are drugs and therapies you should always have on your person when performing dermal fillers as "just in case" should the worst happen, such as hyaluronidase, nitroglycerine paste and aspirin.

## HYALURONIDASE

Hyaluronidase is an enzyme which dissolves hyaluronic acid, the key constituent in most dermal fillers. It needs to be injected directly into the area suspected of being devoid of arterial blood supply. A standard dose required for lysis of dermal fillers is 200 units. Some practitioners advocate mixing it with lidocaine or normal saline to increase the volume of solution and subsequently create a larger *effective volume*. Once administered, the area should be massaged and observed for one hour. If there is no improvement this may be repeated for three to four cycles. It is worth noting that approximately one in 1,000 people have an allergy to hyaluronidase, and subsequently, a skin test should be performed by injecting four units into the skin and observing for five minutes. Should a wheal appear in the skin then an allergy to hyaluronidase should be suspected. Even if no wheal is apparent, please be mindful that a life-threatening anaphylaxis could still occur after hyaluronidase hypodermolysis.

## NITROGLYCERINE PASTE

At present, the evidence to suggest the use of nitroglycerin paste is contentious at best, and therefore it should only be used if you are confident in your abilities and that you believe it is likely to be of benefit to your patients. Nitroglycerin is a prominent vasodilator, and subsequently, you should administer it with the patient lying down to decrease the risk of collapse due to cerebral or cardiac hypoperfusion. Rubbing a small volume into the affected area should cause blood vessels to dilate and hopefully increase tissue perfusion in the area of impending necrosis. It is also advisable for patients to proceed to use nitroglycerin paste two to three times daily for the next few days whilst you continue to monitor them for necrosis. Advise them that headaches or lightheadedness are common side effects of nitroglycerin treatment, and to stop using it and contact you immediately should they have any significant side effects.

### ASPIRIN

Aspirin prevents platelet aggregation and prevents blood clotting by inhibiting thromboxane A2. It is therefore a useful emergency therapy in the context of impending necrosis and should be given to the patient immediately as long as there are no contraindications. It is currently advised to advise a patient to take 300 mg of aspirin daily for at least seven days pending your continued review. It is also worth writing a letter to their general practitioner to inform them you have given them this advice as they are likely to know the patient's history better than you and be well aware of any potential contraindications.

### FURTHER MANAGEMENT

Once you have administered the initial emergency treatment, then it is your duty to follow the patient up daily to give you the best chance to intercept any necrotic areas forming. It is strongly advisable that should your patient's suspected avascular necrosis worsen in front of you despite your best efforts then refer them to hospital immediately. If on daily review their symptoms do not improve or become worse, it is imperative that they see an experienced plastic or maxillofacial surgeon urgently for surgical intervention. If a necrotic area progresses to develop, a large arterial ulcer will form with a significant risk of infection and scarring. When referring your patient, write a letter outlining the dates of treatment, product and volume used, and which steps you have taken to manage it so far.

## VENOUS OCCLUSION

Arteries are not the only vascular structures susceptible to damage or occlusion from dermal filler treatment. The veins of the face are usually relatively thin, superficial vessels which are all too easily obstructed due to filler administration. As veins drain deoxygenated blood from tissues, areas which are affected by venous occlusion may not develop avascular necrosis directly, but will instead have a constant inflow of oxygenated blood with insufficient drainage away from that region. If you were to imagine filling up a water balloon, the water will flow in with no clear path to escape. As pressure builds up the balloon will stretch initially to compensate for this before bursting when the pressure becomes too great. This concept of progressive pressure increase applies to the tissues of the dermis and epidermis in the context of augmentation with dermal fillers.

## PATHOPHYSIOLOGY OF VENOUS OCCLUSION

As in the preceding example, venous occlusion will result in a constant inflow of blood into an area with insufficient venous drainage. The epidermis, dermis, sub-cutaneous tissues and muscles are relatively elastic and will in the acute phase be able to stretch and compensate for this increased pressure. Patients may initially be asymptomatic; however, over time (usually a few hours), they may notice a dull ache in the region of occlusion with a red or blue hue due to an increased retained volume of blood. Although it may not be initially apparent, at a microscopic level the increased pressure will cause damage to local tissues due to a compressive effect which will subsequently damage fragile structures within the local tissue matrix such as nerves, sweat glands and hair follicles. As this progresses, stronger structures (namely arteries and arterioles) will also become compressed and put a patient at risk of delayed avascular necrosis, which has the same pathophysiology as arterial avascular necrosis. See figure 13.2.

Within the first few hours after a venous occlusive event, patients may notice an area of progressive swelling associated with a dull ache. They may also report the aforementioned red or bluish painless swelling, which is a *key discriminator* from arterial occlusion, which is almost always a painful process. As the venous occlusion continues to progress, local tissues will become further damaged and develop

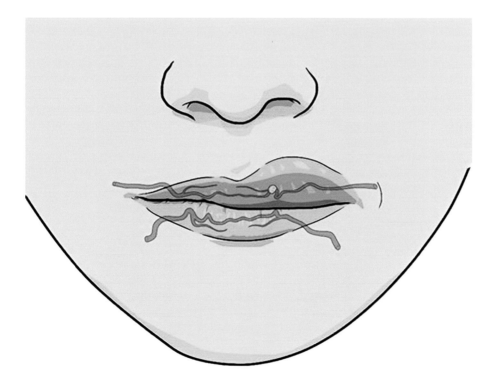

FIGURE 13.2 Diagrammatic representation of venous occlusion.

later stigmata of an occlusive event, such as blistering, pustule formation and tissue necrosis due to local trauma and hypoxia from arterial occlusion.

#### DECREASING THE RISK OF VENOUS OCCLUSION

The same risk stratification methods for arterial occlusion apply to venous occlusion: understanding the local anatomy, using the minimal filler possible for the same effective cosmetic effect and always withdrawing your plunger before injecting. For a more in-depth discussion of this, please familiarise yourself with the subsection outlining the risks of avascular necrosis.

#### MANAGEMENT OF VENOUS OCCLUSION

The management of venous occlusion is essentially the same as in that for impending avascular necrosis. The one caveat is that you may be unable to recognise a venous occlusion in the acute phase as it can take several hours for symptoms to become apparent. It is therefore strongly advised to warn patients of the potential signs and symptoms of venous occlusion, such as continued lip swelling, discoloration and a dull ache (but please bear in mind as previously stated that it may be *painless*).

One different strategy for venous occlusion in comparison to arterial occlusion is to relieve the local pressure effects caused by impaired venous drainage. As tissues fill with undrained blood, this compresses upon the arteries and nerves of local tissues with potentially catastrophic results. Therefore, as an emergency measure, the area of clot can be surgically opened (or attempted to be drained with a green needle) to decrease the increased pressure within tissues. This is by no means a definitive treatment, but it may decrease the chance of a localised compartment syndrome secondary to venous occlusion.

Should a patient contact you later with these symptoms, then please arrange for an urgent review. Ideally you should review all your own patients in the event of an emergency or complication. In the unlikely event that you are indisposed, then arrange for them to see an experienced cosmetic practitioner or plastic surgeon immediately. Do not rely on them to make these arrangements as they may already be distressed and not fully understand the gravity of the situation.

## POST-PROCEDURE INFECTION

There are many factors which can determine the chance of a patient developing a post-procedural infection which are intimately linked with one another creating an overall risk of the probability of infection formation. Some of the key factors to consider are local microbiota, procedural technique and the patient's underlying immunocompetency. Bear all three of these in mind when treating a patient to do your utmost to decrease the chance of a potentially disfiguring infection taking hold.

#### SKIN COMMENSALS

Our skin is home to millions of bacteria which normally cause us no bother whatsoever as long as *they stay there*. Bacteria which naturally live on (or within) us and cause us no

**TABLE 13.1**
**Skin Commensals**

| Bacterial Species | Frequency |
| --- | --- |
| Staphyloccus epidermis | Common |
| Corynebacterium spp | Fairly common |
| Acinetobacter johnsonii | Fairly common |
| Propioniobacterium acnes | Fairly common |
| Streptococcus mitis | Fairly common |
| Staphylococcus aureus | Relatively uncommon |
| Staphylococcus warneri | Relatively uncommon |
| Pseudomonus aeruginosa | Relatively uncommon |
| Streptococcus pyogenes | Relatively uncommon |

harm are known as *commensals*. These microbes play a key role in normal physiological functions such as digestion as well as outcompeting the "bad" bacteria which may cause illness. The flora residing atop the skin differs between regions of our body, much like different species of animals being found in the arctic permafrost to the rainforests of Brazil. We shan't dwell too much on commensals commonly found crawling between our toes (such as the fungus *Candida albicans*) as we are unlikely to be augmenting that region with dermal fillers or botulinum toxin. It is worthwhile understanding the more common bacteria to be found on the face and within the mouth as they are the bugs you are more likely to encounter whilst performing cosmetic treatments. With regards to treating the face, one key feature which influences the skin microbiota here is the relative high density of sebaceous glands, which encourages the growth of lipophilic microorganisms such as *Propionibacterium* spp. and *Malassezia* spp.

Bacteria such as *Staphylococcus aureus* and *Pseudomonas aeruginosa* are just two examples of the many species which can be found living on our skin. These bacteria are unlikely to cause a person harm unless they find themselves *within* the epidermal layer. This is where the primary risk of infection presents itself regarding dermal filler injection. As we are intentionally breaking the skin with a needle in order to perform augmentation, it means that there is a chance of directly inoculating the subcutaneous tissues with both dermal filler and bacteria.

Once the bacteria find themselves within the skin, our immune system recognises them as alien cells due to proteins and metabolites not normally found within eukaryotic cells. Once this has occurred, white blood cells trigger a localised inflammatory response characterised by pain, heat, swelling and erythema which one would easily identify as an infection.

## Risk factors

There are two primary factors which come into play in a post-procedural infection. The first is the pathogens which find themselves within our soft tissues, and the second is patient factors which may make them more susceptible to an infection taking hold. Risk factors can be broken down into local and systemic risk factors for infection.

Regarding a pathogen, the two key factors to consider regarding the chance of them causing an infection are

1. the *volume* of pathogen inoculated and
2. the *virulence* of the pathogen itself.

Simply put, if you introduce a large volume of particularly aggressive pathogens then you are more likely to cause an infection than if you inject a small volume of a more benign microorganism. Due to this, there are several contraindications to dermal filler augmentation regarding localised infection (or potential infection). Such contraindications can be broken down into three main categories:

1. Active skin infection at the proposed injection site (cold sore, warts, cellulitis)
2. Active infection local to the injection site (dental abscess, nasal infection, infective sinusitis, tonsillitis, ear infection etc.)
3. Active systemic infection (gastroenteritis, lower respiratory tract infection, glandular fever, tuberculosis etc.)

Any of these contraindications can be further broken down into bacterial, viral and fungal infections, each with its own presentation, natural history and treatment strategies.

### Bacterial skin infections

Bacterial skin infections are surprisingly common, affecting slightly more than one in every 50 people at some point in their lives. For a bacterial infection to take hold, three distinct processes must occur:

1. Bacterial adherence to host cells
2. Invasion of tissues
3. Toxin release

Of these three processes, it is the release of toxins which arguably contributes the most to the clinical sequelae of a bacterial infection. Bacterial toxins can be classified as either endo- or exotoxins depending on their mechanism of action. Endotoxins are lipopolysaccharide chains which are frequently found within the wall of gram-negative bacteria such as *Pseudomonas aeruginosa*, and in small volumes, they benefit the immune system by acting as potent chemoattractants and costimulators to T-lymphocyte activation. If these lipopolysaccharides are present in large volumes, either due to a particularly virulent strain or a large bacterial load, then this may result in overstimulation of the immune and inflammatory responses. The consequences of a massive inflammatory response include potentially fatal events such as septic shock, disseminated intravascular coagulation and acute respiratory distress syndrome. Exotoxins are proteins secreted by bacteria which are designed to cause tissue damage or disruption through processes such as interrupted enzymatic reactions,

**TABLE 13.2**
**Common Bacterial Skin Infections of the Face**

| Disease | Causative Organism(s) | Clinical Findings | Treatment |
| --- | --- | --- | --- |
| Impetigo | *Staphyloccus aureus* *Streptococcus pyogenes* | Common in children Highly contagious Yellow, potentially itchy crusty lesions May have a bullous form, predominantly caused by *S. aureus* with bullae rupturing to reveal a brown crust | If in a small area, it is usually treated with topical fusidic acid or mupirocin Larger areas are often treated with oral antibiotics such as flucloxacillin or erythromycin |
| Cellulitis | *Staphyloccus aureus* *Streptococcus pyogenes* | Spreading, warm, erythematous area Tender to touch May be systemically unwell | Usually requires antibiotic therapy, PO if stable or IV if systemically unwell Common first-line antibiotics are flucloxacillin or erythromycin |
| Erysipelas | *Streptococcus pyogenes* | Fevers, rigors, systemic upset Erythematous superficial patch extending rapidly with a sharply demarcated, raised edge May weep serious fluid but not pus Peau d'orange may be present Severe infections may have a herpetic or blistering appearance | Usually requires antibiotic therapy, PO if stable or IV if systemically unwell Common first-line antibiotics are flucloxacillin or erythromycin |
| Boils/ Carbuncles | May be any skin commensal, frequently *Staphylococcus spp.* | Tender, painful, erythematous lump Frequently found in hairier/shaved areas Patient usually systemically well | Frequently incision and drainage alone are sufficient Antibiotics are usually only advised if spreading infection or systemically unwell |
| Folliculitis | *Staphyloccus aureus* *Pseudomonas aeruginosa* | Crop of pustules in moist, hairy area May be tender or itchy May be associated with hot tub/sauna use | Usually none required If symptomatic, consider topical fusidic acid or mupirocin to start |

cellular dysregulation or pore formation. All three processes have the same overall objective: cell death. The induction of cell lysis by exotoxins is an evolutionary function developed by bacteria in order for them to carve out a niche environment within the host for them to propagate further. One particularly unpleasant category of exotoxins are *superantigens*, secreted by bacteria such as *Staphylococcus aureus* and *Streptococcus pyogenes*. These antigens bind to T-lymphocyte receptors and stimulate a massive, yet poorly regulated inflammatory response. The consequence of this is significant tissue necrosis, thus helping the bacteria to create a new home within their host. Superantigen secretion is believed to be a key factor in the development and precipitation of toxic shock syndrome.

The response of the body to bacterial infection is to initiate an inflammatory response with the intention of destroying the infection and stimulating the repair of damaged tissues. Inflamed tissues are hyperaemic to allow for increased oxygen and lymphocyte delivery with enhanced venous drainage to remove toxic metabolites. Lymphocytes are attracted to the area of infection by cytokine mediators and on arrival will attack bacteria. The dead bacterial are then phagocytosed and digested by phagocytes. Cytokines released by immune cells, such as tumour necrosis factor (TNF) and interleukins 1 and 6, are mediators in the development of a fever as a response to these infections with the intention of disrupting bacterial enzymatic processes and contributing to their demise.

Table 13.2 gives a selection of common bacterial infections to affect the face, their causative organism and potential treatment options.

## Viral skin infections

Similar to bacterial skin infections, cutaneous viral infections often begin with defects in the skin such as a small abrasion or cut. The predominant difference between viral and bacterial infections is that all viruses are obligatory intracellular parasites: they *cannot* live without an infected host cell to reside within. The main three ways viruses enter host cells are fusion with the plasma membrane of the host cell, being endocytosed or directly injecting the viral capsid or genome into the host. Once the virus has taken hold of the host cell machinery, it hijacks the cellular replication machinery and directs it to instead replicate the virus. When the cell has replicated the virus (this may be millions of times) the host cell dies and the virus is *shedded*, with potentially millions of new viruses being expelled into the local environment propagating the infection as each individual virus tries to replicate the above lifecycle.

Our bodies do not just sit idly by whilst these infections occur, and we have evolved many sophisticated mechanisms in order to impede the progression of a viral infection. One important innate defence against viral infection is a process known as RNA interference. As viruses use cellular replication machinery to propagate their own progeny, cells can utilise a complex protein known as the *RNA-induced silencing complex* to cleave newly formed viral mRNA and prevent translation of the viral genome. Adaptive immunity against viral infections includes the production of antibodies to bind to and incapacitate viral invaders, with IgM produced in the acute phase and IgG conferring lifelong immunity to a specific pathogen. The cellular component of adaptive immunity involves lineages such as cytotoxic T-lymphocytes, which target cells infected cells by recognising viral antigens on their cell surface, binding to these cells and releasing cytotoxins such as perforin, granzymes and granulysin. These cytotoxins induce cell death with the intention of killing the virus through terminating the infected host cell.

There are several viral skin infections; however, the only one which is likely to have an impact on your cosmetic practice is herpes simplex virus (HSV). This virus is responsible for a condition called *Herpes labialis*, colloquially known as a "cold sore". HSV is an incredibly infectious pathogen and is commonly transmitted between individuals through close contact with a person shedding the virus or through mucosal, oral or genital secretions. The virus presents as exquisitely tender intraepidermal vesicles which frequently rupture and crust after two to three days of onset with persistent sores, blisters or crusting afterwards. Symptoms often subside within two weeks of onset, yet the virus is not eradicated from the body but lays dormant within the ganglion of the trigeminal nerve. Patients with HSV infection may experience flares of the condition precipitated by sunlight, menstruation, local trauma, illness and stress. As herpes labialis is believed to affect between one quarter and one third of young people and a flare can be precipitated by stress or local trauma, it should be a key consideration in the context of lip augmentation. Specifically ask your patients if they have a history of cold sores or if they have recently been in close contact with a person with one. Advise your patient that proceeding with treatment may induce a flare of their herpes labialis. It is worth noting, however, that most cases do not require any specific treatment bar supportive care. Parenteral antivirals are usually only reserved for patients at risk of developing systemic herpes infection; however, some practitioners advocate the use or oral or topical acyclovir when treating patients with a history of cold sores to prevent a flare.

## Fungal skin infections

Fungal skin infections on the whole are relatively common; however, relatively few affect the skin of the face. Most fungi exhibit a preference for warm, moist areas such as oral mucosa or creases in the groin. Fungal infections of the skin can be divided in respect to their depth, classified as either superficial mycoses affecting the outer epidermis or hair; cutaneous mycoses of the deep epidermis and hair follicles or nails; and subcutaneous mycoses of the fat, muscle and fascia. Of these three superficial and cutaneous mycoses are by far the most common. Systemic fungal infections are rare unless a person is immunocompromised, which we shall explain in more detail later in this chapter. Other important risk factors for a fungal infection include poor hygiene, damage to mucosal barriers and the recent use of antibiotics.

Fungi are fascinating microbes in that they display microscopic features of both animal and plant cells (such as a membrane-bound nucleus and cell wall) and subsequently have their own kingdom for classification purposes. The most common species of fungi are *Aspergillus* and *Candida*, and despite being recognised commensals they also are responsible for potentially serious infections, with *Aspergillus* being responsible for aspergillosis and *Candida* responsible for a condition colloquially known as thrush.

*Dermatophytes* are arguably the commonest cause of fungal skin infections, and they include pathogens such as *Trichophyton* and *Microsporum* genera, causing conditions such as tinea capitis and tinea faciei. Non-dermatophytes also play a role, with fungi such as *Malassezia globosa*, and *Candida albicans* cause conditions such as pityriasis versicolor, cutaneous candidiasis, respectively.

Dermatophyte infections commonly present as asymmetrical erythematous, scaly well-demarcated patches which may or may not be pruritic in nature. Patients will inform you that these patches are slow-growing, with an erythematous scaly ring. Do not be surprised if there is also a relatively well-preserved central area. There may be associated well-defined patchy hair loss in regions affected with dermatophyte infections, which is frequently and unsurprisingly upsetting for patients. These infections are usually easily treated with topical antifungal agents such as cotrimazole cream.

## PATIENT FACTORS IN DEVELOPING INFECTION

Our bodies are under a near-constant attack from opportunistic pathogens which could potentially cause us serious harm. Fortunately, to combat this, we have our immune system, comprised of nonspecific, primitive and inaccurate *innate immunity* and more refined, targeted *adaptive immunity*. These two systems work in conjunction with one another to help prevent infectious diseases taking hold.

### INNATE IMMUNITY: SKIN, MUCOUS MEMBRANES AND BODILY FLUIDS

Innate immunity is the body's first line of defence to external pathogens. This is an imprecise process and cannot identify specific pathogens for targeted destruction. Components of the innate immune system include chemical and physical barriers provided by the skin and mucous membranes as well as internal defences, such as antimicrobial substances; cells, such as natural killer cells and phagocytes; and the inflammatory response composed of both inflammation and pyrexia.

The primary defence of the body to external pathogens are the skin and mucous membranes, which provide both physical and chemical barriers to impede microbes from entering and causing disease. The tough and tightly bound keratinised outer layer of the epidermis provides a stern mechanical barricade to foreign cells, as well as shedding keratinocytes periodically to remove surface microbes. It is highly unlikely that bacteria, viruses or fungi will be able to penetrate the epidermal layer in an immunocompetent individual unless it is damaged through burns or cuts in the skin.

Internally, epithelial cells within the mucous membranes secrete mucous, a sticky substance which functions to both lubricate and moisturise the surfaces of body cavities. As it is both thick and sticky, mucous can also trap pathogens, halting their invasion attempts. Within the respiratory tract, these epithelial linings have specialised projections called *cilia*, which beat continuously and in unison away from the lungs. The function of cilia is to manoeuvre mucous out of the lower respiratory tract towards the mouth where it can be expelled via a cough or a sneeze; or swallowed and digested by the stomach. This process is designed to destroy potentially harmful microbes; however, it can inadvertently offer a method of disease progression through aerosol droplets. It is worth noting that certain diseases can result in impaired mucous and cilia function, namely cystic fibrosis (which causes excessively thick mucous production) and Kartagener's syndrome, characterised by dysregulated cilia motion.

Aside from mucous, there are other important bodily fluids which protect an individual from infection:

- Tears produced by the lacrimal glands which both dilute microbes and contain an enzyme called lysozyme which can digest bacterial cell walls
- Saliva which washes bacteria from the oral cavity and maintains a normal pH
- Urine expelling bacteria from the urinary tract
- Sebum produced by sebaceous glands in the skin inhibiting the growth of certain bacteria and fungi
- Gastric acid produced by parietal cells in the stomach maintain an acid environment, which is hostile to most microbiota
- Vaginal secretions to prevent epithelial tissue breakdown and expel bacteria

It is worth noting, however, that most fluid secretions only offer immunity should they continue to *flow*. Stasis of any of the previously mentioned bodily fluids can allow them to stagnate and afford a potential niche for bacteria or fungi to take hold.

### INNATE IMMUNITY: INTERNAL ANTIMICROBIAL STRATEGIES

Should the external barriers to the body be breached by microbes, the next line of defence of the innate immune system is activated. The functions of this aspect of the innate immune system are varied, complex and very effective. Internal antimicrobial strategies include the production of antimicrobial substances, innate immune cells, inflammation, and pyrexia.

### ANTIMICROBIAL SUBSTANCES

There are four key antimicrobial substances which are involved in internal microbial defence: interferons, complement proteins, iron-binding proteins and antimicrobial proteins. *Interferons* (IFNs) are signalling proteins expressed by lymphocytes, macrophages, and fibroblasts after they have been infected with an intracellular pathogen, such as a virus. By expressing interferons, these cells are able to flag themselves up for destruction by natural killer cells and macrophages, as well as acting as an early warning system for nearby cells that a microbial attack is underway. This process allows local cells to take certain steps to prevent viral replication, such as the production of enzymes which destroy RNA or inhibit protein synthesis. The first step in interferon production is the identification of *foreign* molecules such as viral RNA or bacterial endotoxins by specialised proteins called *pattern recognition receptors*. Once activated, these receptors initiate the production of interferons such as IFN-$\alpha$, IFN-$\gamma$ and NF-K$\beta$ which result in an amplified immune response via downstream signalling through transcription factors such as signal transducer and activation of transcription (STAT) complex.

STAT complexes amplify the immune response by selectively upregulating certain genes involved in the immune system with subsequent increased production of antimicrobial proteins. Further interferon functions include the upregulation of *major histocompatibility complexes* (MHC) which increase the exposure of viral proteins to cytotoxic and helper T-lymphocytes for improved recognition of infected cells and the production of pro-inflammatory cytokines and the direct activation of both natural killer cells and macrophages.

*The complement system* is comprised of approximately thirty proteins which are synthesised by the liver and are permanently in circulation in blood plasma. When complement proteins are triggered by microbial antigens, a cascade of events is initiated with the intention of destroying pathogens through phagocytosis, cytolysis and inflammation. Phagocytosis is triggered via a process called *opsonisation*, where opsonin proteins are used to mark infected or dying cells to be phagocytosed. Cytolysis occurs through the formation of the membrane attack complex (MAC) which effectively punches a hole within the plasma membrane of bacteria, causing them to rupture due to an inflow of extracellular fluid. Finally, inflammation is stimulated by the binding of complement proteins to mast cells to encourage them to secrete histamine which increases blood vessel permeability to allow cells of the immune system to extravasate and reach the target area.

The cascading nature of complement protein activation allows for rapid amplification of a signal, and therefore a trace amount of pathogenic material can result in a large and coordinated immune response. There are three main ways in which the complement cascade can be activated:

1. *The classical pathway* occurs when IgG or IgM antibodies bind to and form a complex with microbial antigens with resultant phagocytosis, cytolysis and inflammation.
2. *The alternative pathway* does not rely on antibodies but instead is triggered by interactions between lipid-carbohydrate complexes on the surface of microbes.
3. *The lectin pathway* is initiated when macrophages digest microbes and release chemicals which stimulate the liver to produce proteins called lectins which bind to carbohydrates on the surface of microbes.

All three of the preceding pathways can initiate the complement cascade; however, they are not independent entities and all three may be activated independently of one another at various stages of the immune response to infection.

*Iron-binding proteins* directly inhibit bacterial growth by decreasing the amount of available iron, with examples including transferrin, lactoferrin, ferritin and haemoglobin. This is why ferritin may be considered an acute-phase protein, with higher-than-expected circulating levels in the setting of acute infection. Iron is required almost universally by all known human pathogens for cellular functions such as DNA replication and respiration. Due to this, the human body has evolved to tightly regulate the amount of freely available iron, allowing it to starve pathogens of this precious resource. One key molecule in iron regulation is the hormone *hepcidin*, which functions by preventing the release of iron from intracellular stores into the systemic circulation through the iron export channel *ferroportin*. By keeping iron within cells, bacteria are unable to access it and their cellular processes are inhibited.

*Antimicrobial peptides* (AMPs) are short peptides which have a wide scope of antimicrobial activity, with some being directly toxic and others attracting dendritic and mast cells to potentiate immune responses. These peptides are ancient and well-preserved throughout both eukaryotic and prokaryotic cells. One particularly important and well-studied family of AMPs are *defensins*, which are expressed by epithelial cells and leukocytes, as well as within breast milk and thus offer a key role in neonatal immunity and function by altering the ionic gradient across bacterial cell membranes by having a higher affinity for ions such as $Ca^{2+}$ and $Mg^{2+}$. Altering the ionic gradient across the plasma membrane causes membrane instability, pore complex formation, membrane depolarisation and finally cell lysis.

## NATURAL KILLER CELLS AND PHAGOCYTES

These cell lines offer a nonspecific, cell-mediated form of defence against microbial pathogens and can be found circulating in blood plasma as well as within the spleen, red bone marrow and lymph nodes. Natural killer (NK) cells can target a plethora of infected human cell lines as well as cells which have become cancerous, provided they express protein signalling molecules identifying them for destruction. Once an NK cell has bound to a target cell, cytotoxic substances are released to destroy them. These substances include perforin proteins which insert into the plasma membrane, creating channels between the cell cytoplasm and the local environment (the name perforin derives from their *function* – to perforate cell membranes). The pores created by perforin proteins allow extracellular fluid to flow into the cell due to a difference in osmotic pressure, and eventually these cells become so engorged with extracellular fluid they pop. Another method of cellular destruction employed by NK cells is through the use of a family of enzymes called *granzymes*. Granzymes destroy intracellular protein, forcing the host cell to undergo apoptosis due to disrupted cellular metabolism. NK cells are a blunt tool, and there is an evolutionary flaw in their function: they do not actually *kill* bacteria within host cells; they merely take away the host in which they reside. Admittedly, some bacteria will inevitably be destroyed as collateral damage from cytolysis, many more will be released into the local environment unscathed. Fortunately, the innate immunity has a back-up plan to address this issue in the form of another specialised cell line called *phagocytes*.

Phagocytes are a family of cells comprised of macrophages and neutrophils which engulf and digest microbes and cellular debris. By digesting unwanted bacteria and debris, the surrounding environment can be cleansed to allow for the eradication of infection and proper wound healing. Infections cause the release of cytokines which attract phagocytes to the affected area. As they migrate, macrophages differentiate and change their behaviour, some become *wandering macrophages* that become larger and begin to hunt down pathogens and toxic debris, whereas other macrophages will become *fixed macrophages* and stand guard within specific tissues to anticipate any potential spread of infection. Alongside their direct role in removing harmful pathogens and material from an area of infection, macrophages also play a key role in mediating inflammation and wound healing, as discussed previously.

The innate immune system is an ancient and effective method of defending us from potentially life-threatening diseases; however, as previously discussed, it is a blunt instrument at best. One key flaw with innate immunity is that it does not improve with successive exposures; simply put, it will mount an almost identical response regardless of how many times it faces the same pathogen. The innate immune system, however, is far more intelligent and will learn to identify pathogens and target them with precision, frequently preventing them from causing us serious harm. There are two key pathways of defence in the adaptive immune system, and these are cell-mediated and antibody-mediated immunity, two complex and interlinked strategies to mount an effective defence versus pathogenic organisms.

*Cell-mediated immunity* is tremendously effective against intracellular pathogens, cancers and parasites. There are two primary cell lines: T and B lymphocytes, with the letter of their name determining where they mature—with T lymphocytes (composed of T-helper and T-cytotoxic lymphocytes) maturing in the thymus and B lymphocytes maturing in red bone marrow. A key step in the maturation process is the development of plasma membrane proteins known as antigen receptors that identify *specific* antigens to allow for a focused attack. The process of maturation allows cells to develop *immunocompetence*—the ability to defend us from infections without inadvertently attacking our own cells with their cytotoxic mediators.

When we are born, our adaptive immune system is relatively weak due to a lack of exposure to pathogenic antigens. Once we have sustained an exposure, antigens are shown to T and B lymphocytes to allow them to recognise the antigens as harmful. These cells then replicate to create an army of specially trained lymphocytes which are able to identify and destroy invading microbes. Some cells remain within the thymus and red bone marrow (memory T and B lymphocytes, respectively) which function to educate naïve lymphocytes in identifying these specific pathogens to allow for an attack in the future. See Figure 13.3.

Most T lymphocytes are inactive the majority of the time and float around in plasma anticipating microbial invasion. So as to not become accidentally activated, these cells require two separate stimuli for activation to occur. The first stimulus is usually the binding of an antigen to T-cell receptors, and the second is a pro-inflammatory cytokine giving them the green light to attack. By lying dormant for significant periods of time, inadvertent damage to our own tissues is reduced, as well as prolonging the life span of T lymphocytes with a greater probability of them being present in significant numbers when required.

Cytotoxic T lymphocytes can be perceived as the assassins of the immunological world. Once activated, they will target and destroy cells infected with a *specific* pathogen. The previously discussed NK cells can target a wide range of infected cells, whereas cytotoxic T lymphocytes will only attack cells infected with pathogens they recognise. Their method of destroying infected cells is relatively similar to NK cells, with the insertion of perforin proteins, as well as pumping toxic chemicals such as granulysin and lymphotoxin to induce apoptosis within the target cell. To ensure that rogue antigens and escaping microbes are not allowed to wreak

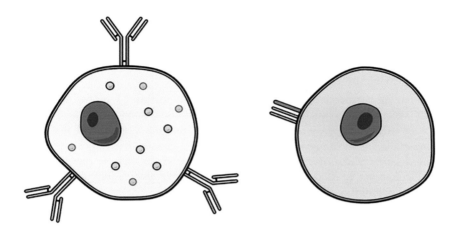

**FIGURE 13.3**   Diagrammatic representation of a T lymphocyte (left) and a B lymphocyte (right).

havoc elsewhere, cytotoxic T lymphocytes secrete IFN-γ, which attracts and activates phagocytes as well as macrophage migration factor to keep them at the site of infection where they are required most.

*Antibody-mediated immunity* is controlled primarily by B lymphocytes. If we are to consider NK cells, phagocytes and T lymphocytes as the front-line soldiers of the immune system, it is pertinent to think of B lymphocytes as the generals who coordinate and amplify the attack itself. When microbes invade our body, the front-line cells race to the site of infection to begin to fight it off, whereas B-lymphocytes remain within lymphoid organs awaiting activation by specific antigens. When antigens reach B-lymphocytes, they are absorbed and processed with the encouragement of nearby T-helper lymphocytes. Once they have absorbed and processed antigens (with co-stimulation from T-helper lymphocytes), B-lymphocytes become active and differentiate into plasma cells and memory B-lymphocytes. Plasma cells secrete millions of antibodies specific to the antigen in question for up to five days after activation after which they die, whereas memory B lymphocytes remain within the red bone marrow where they can differentiate into new plasma cells and memory B lymphocytes should there be another infection from the same pathogen.

Antibodies aid the immune response through a series of separate functions:

- Neutralisation of antigens and bacterial toxins by binding to them and rendering them inactive. They also offer some protection in inhibiting viral attachment to host cells.
- Sticking multiple antigens together in a process called agglutination, forming a ball of inactive antigens which are easily phagocytosed
- Stimulating phagocytosis by acting as cell-signalling molecules and upregulating the activity of phagocytic cells

- Activating the complement cascade
- Attacking cilia and flagella of bacteria, immobilising them and thus preventing their spread and making them easier targets for destruction

## IMMUNODEFICIENCY DISORDERS

From a patient perspective, the primary factor in determining whether they will or will not succumb to a post-procedural infection is their immune status. There are two main ways a person will have a weakened immune system, and that is usually due to a *primary immunodeficiency disorder* (a genetic disease) or a *secondary immunodeficiency disorder*, an acquired condition which may be due to diseases such as leukaemia, or secondary to immunosuppressive medications started by doctors with the *intention* of dampening a patient's immune system, such as steroid use in the context of inflammatory arthritides.

### PRIMARY IMMUNODEFICIENCY DISORDERS

Primary immunodeficiency disorders (PIDs) arise from genetic mutations and are present from birth. At the time of publishing, there are more than 300 recognised PIDs, with an incidence of approximately between one in 500 and one in 1200 live births. The human immune system is a multifaceted and complex system, and genetic mutations causing PIDs can affect any of the steps involved in mounting an appropriate immune response, including both the innate and adaptive immune systems. Table 13.3 has a table of some of the more common PIDs and which areas of the immune system are compromised in them.

## TABLE 13.3
## Primary Immunodeficiency Disorders

| Condition | Mutation | Effect on Immunity |
|---|---|---|
| *Selective IgA Deficiency* | Mutations in chromosomes 6, 14 & 18 | B Lymphocytes are unable to produce IgA, resulting in immunocompromise of mucous membranes |
| *Common Variable Immunodeficiency* | Poorly understood. Believed to be mutations in ICOS, TACI, CD 19/20/21/80 and BAFFR genes | Low circulating immunoglobulins (primarily IgG, IgM and IgA) |
| *Severe Combined Immunodeficiency* | CD132 gene (X Chromosome) | Impaired production of IL-2, IL-4, IL-7, IL-9, IL-15 and IL-21, resulting in a lack of differentiation and maturation of T and B lymphocytes |
| *X-Linked Agammaglobulinaemia* | Btk gene (X Chromosome) | No gamma globulin production with subsequent lack of mature B-lymphocyte production |

**TABLE 13.3  (Continued)**

| Condition | Mutation | Effect on Immunity |
|---|---|---|
| *Wiskott-Aldrich Syndrome* | WAS gene (X Chromosome) | Impaired lymphocyte and platelet cytoskeleton development, making a person susceptible to bleeding and infections |
| *DiGeorge Syndrome* | Deletion of genes at 22q11.2 (Chromosome 22) | Thymic hypoplasia with resultant lack of T-cell maturation |
| *Louis-Bar Syndrome* | ATM Gene (Chromosome 11) | Low IgA and IgG levels (IgM can be high or low). Low CD4 count. Impaired lymphoid cell survival |

Selective IgA deficiency is one of the more common PIDs, and as approximately 1 in 600 people are born with this condition, there is a chance you may come across a person with it during your cosmetic practice. Due to it weakening the immune response of mucous membranes, it puts patients at a heightened risk of infection, particularly after perioral or perinasal augmentation.

SECONDARY IMMUNODEFICIENCY DISORDERS

Secondary immunodeficiency disorders (SIDs) are acquired during a person's life. They can be further subdivided into medical or physical conditions which dampen the immune system as well as iatrogenic immunodeficiency due to medical therapies (Tables 13.4 and 13.5). SIDs are vastly more common than PIDs, and subsequently, you must have a good awareness of associated conditions to ensure safe practice. One example of a

**TABLE 13.4**
**A Selection of Conditions Causing Secondary Immune Deficiency**

| Condition | Signs & Symptoms | Effect on Immune System |
|---|---|---|
| Diabetes mellitus | Fatigue, polyuria, polydipsia, confusion, mood swings, coma | Decreased chemotaxis, adherence and phagocytosis by neutrophils. Decreased differentiation into macrophages. impaired activation of complement cascade. |
| HIV/AIDS | Fatigue, weight loss, repeated infections | Decreased CD4 (T-helper cell) count leads to reversal of CD4:CD8 ratio and subsequent immunosuppression. |
| Malnutrition (note this can be due to under- or over-nutrition) | Weight loss/gain, loss of hair and teeth, fatigue, dizziness | Decreased innate and adaptive immune function (decreased IgA/B-cell count, lymphocyte hypo-responsiveness) |
| Metastatic malignancy | History of malignancy. Bony "toothache pain". May keep them up at night. Loss of height. Unprovoked fracture | Decreased bone marrow production of white blood cells |

*(Continued)*

## TABLE 13.4 (Continued)

| Condition | Signs & Symptoms | Effect on Immune System |
|---|---|---|
| Haematological malignancy | Night sweats, weight loss, fatigue, swollen lymph nodes, abdominal discomfort | White blood cells may be poorly differentiated/functioning |
| Bone marrow disorder (e.g. myelofibrosis) | Fatigue, shortness of breath, easy bruising, easy bleeding, night sweats | Decreased bone marrow production of white blood cells |
| Chronic kidney disease | Oedema, fatigue, weight loss, poor appetite | Downregulation of B cells, decreased bactericidal abilities of monocytes |
| Splenectomy | History of splenectomy! (Usually secondary to trauma | Low circulating concentrations of IgM, decreased circulating T cells and reduced lymphocyte proliferative responses |
| Haemoglobulinopathies (e.g. Thalassamia) | Fatigue, jaundice, abdominal fullness, dark urine | Decreased B- and T-cell function, decreased immunoglobulin production |

## TABLE 13.5
## Immunosuppressive Medications

| Drug | Indication | Effect on Immune System |
|---|---|---|
| Ciclosporin | Prevention of graft versus host disease | Reversibly inhibits cell-mediated and antibody-specific immune responses |
| Azathioprine | Prevention of graft versus host disease. Also used in autoimmune conditions where corticosteroid therapy alone is inadequate | Impairs DNA synthesis and results in death of rapidly dividing cells |
| Methotrexate | Rheumatoid arthritis, chemotherapy, psoriasis, Crohn's disease | Inhibits T-cell activation, suppresses intracellular adhesion molecules of T cell, selectively downregulated B cells |
| Glucocorticoids | Replacement of endogenous corticosteroids, rheumatoid arthritis, inflammatory bowel disease, asthma | Decreased production and function of T and B cells. Inhibition of the complement cascade |
| Mycophenolate Mofetil | Used alongside corticosteroids and ciclosporin to prevent acute transplant rejection | Impairs T and B cell proliferation |

particularly common secondary immunodeficiency disorder is type II diabetes mellitus (TIIDM), a condition which affects approximately one in sixteen people in the United Kingdom. By understanding the way in which conditions such as TIIDM dampen a person's immune system, you will be able to properly counsel patients with these conditions to allow them to achieve informed consent before initiating a procedure.

So as to not become too confusing, we shall break down SIDs into "Conditions" and "Medications". By understanding which conditions can predispose somebody to immunodeficiency and a few cardinal signs and symptoms in the case of the as-yet undiagnosed, you will be able to both properly assess and consent a patient for treatment. Similarly to medical conditions, it is also important to understand the indications and pharmacology of immunosuppressive medications so you don't inadvertently treat an immunosuppressed individual and put them at undue risk.

SIGNS AND SYMPTOMS OF INFECTION

Infections and inflammatory conditions are characterised primarily by four primary symptoms:

1. *Dolor* (pain)
2. *Rubor* (erythema)
3. *Calor* (heat)
4. *Tumor* (swelling)

Look out for all of these if a patient presents to you with what may be an infection. Take the time to properly assess the injection site and area surrounding it for pain, erythema, heat and swelling. Ask your patient if where you are pressing is painful, and when they first noticed the symptoms. It may take a few days for an infection to take hold and become symptomatic, especially if they have been taking paracetamol or ibuprofen to help them with the initial post-procedural discomfort. If a patient calls you under 24 hours after a treatment reporting these symptoms, infection is a less likely cause as it is unlikely to present clinically within this time frame, yet it is still important to assess them and keep infection as a possible differential diagnosis.

Sometimes simply lymphadenopathy may be the first presentation of an infective process. Fortunately, due to their relatively predictable drainage patterns, it is often possible to "track back" along the route of lymphatics to try to identify the infective focus. Do not forget that painful lymphadenopathy is often associated with infection or inflammation, yet painless lymphadenopathy should raise clinical suspicion

**TABLE 13.6**
**Lymphatic Drainage of the Face**

| Lymph Nodes | Location | Drains |
|---|---|---|
| Infraorbital | Nasolabial fold | Medial eyelid, canthus, nose |
| Buccinator | Angle of the mouth | Lower eyelid, cheek, temporal region |
| Mandibular | Anterior to masseter | Cheeks and lower lips |
| Malar | Zygomatic arch | Eyelids, lateral canthus, temporal region |
| Superficial extrafacial | Anterior to tragus | Forehead, temporal region, root of nose, pinna |
| Pre-auricular | Anterior to tragus | Forehead, temporal region, root of nose, pinna |
| Infra-auricular | Between inferior border of parotid and anterior border of sternocleidomastoid | Posterior cheek, nose, upper eyelid. |
| Deep intraglandular | Within the parotid gland | Forehead, temporal region, lateral eyelid, lacrimal gland, external and middle ear |

for a malignant process. As a brief aide memoire, Table 13.6 outlines the expected lymphatic drainage from structures pertinent to facial aesthetics, outlining their anatomical considerations as discussed in Chapter 3.

## ABSCESSES

Infections, particularly those bacterial in origin, may develop into abscesses. An abscess is a collection of pus surrounded by a wall of granulation tissue, and on examination you may well be able to palpate a fluctuant lump. This is likely to be warm to the touch and exquisitely tender for the patient when palpated. Patients with an abscess may also commonly report *swinging pyrexias*, high temperatures which come and go in a cyclical manner. Therefore, should a patient comes to you with reporting these symptoms in the area treated after filler augmentation, then an abscess should be your primary differential. Maintain a high index of suspicion for this and arrange for urgent treatment.

Please note: for discussion of cellulitis, please refer to the relevant section in Chapter 10.

### MANAGEMENT OF AN ABSCESS

An abscess is a collection of pus formed within a cavity in soft tissues created by bacterial infection. Bacteria release toxic mediators which cause necrosis of surrounding cells. As we discussed previously regarding avascular necrosis, whilst T and B cells invade the area of necrotic tissue to fight off the infection, cells in the periphery undergo apoptosis to form a perimeter around the area of necrosis to prevent its continued and unregulated spread. As part of the inflammatory response, pro-inflammatory cytokines such as IL-6, IL-10 and TNF-$\alpha$ are released by immune cells which protracts pain, erythema and swelling of local tissues. The pus within the abscess cavity is composed of tissue debris, dead cells, white blood cells and extracellular fluid.

The management of abscesses has been documented for millennia, and there is even a phrase in Latin for it: *Ubi pus, ibi evacua*! This, for the non-Latin scholars amongst you, means "Where [there is pus], there evacuate [it]". Abscesses in the context of dermal filler injection may present primarily in one of two ways: a localised hot, red, angry and fluctuant lump is likely secondary to direct inoculation of a skin commensal to the subcutaneous tissues, whereas if the entire area treated forms an abscess in the acute phase, then it is worth bearing in mind that it may be an infected batch of dermal filler instead. One of the concerns with an abscess formation after dermal filler augmentation is that you have not only introduced infection but also a hyaluronic acid gel for pathogens to develop within. By introducing infection and a glycosaminoglycan simultaneously, the bacteria will effectively be delivered in a "grow-bag" to allow them to flourish in their new environment, potentially making drainage and definitive treatment of an abscess after dermal filler augmentation more difficult than an uncomplicated skin abscess.

Abscesses demand urgent and definitive management. Your first step should be aspirating the abscess to get a sample for microscopy and culture by a microbiologist. Inflamed skin can be notoriously difficult to anaesthetise due to the increased acidity of tissues; therefore (if you are suitably trained and comfortable to do so), a dental block may sufficiently anaesthetise your patient before aspirating or incising a lip abscess.

Aspirate as much pus as you can as this will have a not only diagnostic benefit but also a therapeutic one (as your patient will be feeling much better once it is drained).

After you have drained the abscess, start the patient on high-dose broad-spectrum antibiotics (such as clindamycin) and ensure that you have sufficient anaerobic cover. Some clinicians also advise the use of hyaluronidase in the event of abscess formation to degrade the filler in situ.

Ensure they have suitable analgesia as abscesses are notoriously painful. Arrange to see them daily, and if you have any suspicion that your management isn't working, or if they become progressively unwell then refer them urgently to an experienced plastic or maxillofacial surgeon as they may require surgical drainage. Yet again write them a letter with information on which product you used, the volume, when you treated the patient and which steps you have taken to treat the abscess thus far. As in the case of cellulitis, ensure you inform your product manufacturer with the batch number of the product used.

## OVERFILLING

Inserting too much filler into an area is an easy mistake to make, especially when you are starting your practice and aren't subconsciously aware of the pressure required to introduce dermal filler into a specific tissue plane. Overfilling is usually more noticeable when treating the lips due to a paucity of overlying subcutaneous fat and connective tissue. The risks of overfilling are not simply limited to an undesirable cosmetic outcome but may also predispose to vascular occlusion and infection.

Identifying an overfilled area at the time of treatment may be difficult due to localised swelling caused by filler administration. If you are confident that you have indeed inserted too much filler into an area, the first thing you need to do is inform your patient. Be honest with them and let them know what has happened and how you intend to fix it. This will decrease confusion on their part when you begin taking the necessary steps to treat it, allowing for informed consent and upholding your duty of candour.

The first step to rectifying overfilling is to milk the area you have filled. If it is lips, nasolabial folds or marionette lines then place your thumb within the lip and index finger on the skin and slide them firmly in a distal to proximal direction in relation your injection line to try and squeeze the filler out of your puncture site. If it is a region overlying a bony prominence, such as the cheeks, then just use your thumb and rely on the underlying bone to provide pressure to the deeper aspect of the augmented area whilst you milk out the filler.

A second approach to overfilling is to simply add more filler to the contralateral side. This will be reliant on your cosmetic eye, as it may be that accidentally adding more filler has created a more desirable cosmetic outcome. If this is the case, consent your patient to the addition of extra filler and augment the other side, and warn them that it may actually confer a worsened appearance. This strategy may be more relevant in the instance of lip augmentation, as some patients may want bigger lips than they previously requested. This strategy is best employed when you are more confident in your abilities, ensuring that your patient has given informed consent. It is unwise to merely keep adding filler in the hope of hiding asymmetry if you will create an undesirable cosmetic outcome.

If you do not notice an area of overfilling whilst with the patient, and they contact you to inform you of asymmetry, firstly assess them in person. On examination you may find it is just soft-tissue swelling without excess filler in that region, and you can reassure the patient that it will settle on its own. Yet again you may wish to add a touch of filler to the contralateral side to balance things out, should you and the patient believe it to yield a successful cosmetic outcome. Be wary, however, that an area of swelling post-procedure may be infective in nature, and subsequently, ensure to screen them for the aforementioned signs of infection before proceeding with any further therapy.

Arguably most radical approach to treating an area which has been overfilled with hyaluronic acid is to locally administer hyaluronidase to dissolve the dermal filler. This enzyme will break down hyaluronic acid in tissues and subsequently decrease the volume of hyaluronic acid present. Hyaluronidase therapy can be a risky strategy for two main reasons: *anaphylaxis* and *poor cosmesis*. Hyaluronidase is made from animal derivatives and therefore may induce an allergic reaction, including *life-threatening anaphylactic shock*. The other consideration is that once you have administered it, you have little control as to how much filler (and indeed native hyaluronic acid) it will dissolve. Therefore consent your patient to allergy, anaphylaxis and undesirable cosmesis before proceeding. Frequently they may require further treatments with dermal filler in the future in order to rectify the area which you have dissolved. To decrease the chance of anaphylaxis it is advisable to perform a skin prick test with a tiny dose of hyaluronidase first. Inject a small volume superficially in the arm and monitor it for a few minutes. Should a wheal develop, then it is likely the patient is indeed allergic to hyaluronidase, and therefore, treatment with hyaluronidase is contraindicated. Should they exhibit symptoms of allergy or anaphylaxis (such as itching, wheals, wheezing, or difficulty breathing) during this prick test or after administration then treat swiftly and accordingly as discussed later in this chapter.

One final approach to overfilling is to simply apologise to the patient and undertake a "watch and wait" strategy. If the overfilled area is not causing any significant emotional or physical discomfort and you are confident there is no underlying infection or risk of vascular occlusion, you may wish to simply leave it in situ. There are risks to any intervention you wish to undertake after overfilling, and as fillers are naturally degraded over time, it may be prudent to just monitor the situation and let nature take its course. Some patients will be happy with this approach, and it is your duty to inform them that this is an option before you undertake any further management.

## ACUTE FILLER LUMPS

Lumps and bumps are a common occurrence after dermal filler augmentation. The two most common causes for lump formation are bolusing filler in an inappropriate location and inserting filler too superficially. It is unlikely to be the filler itself which is problematic, other than if you were to use an incorrect viscosity filler within a specific tissue plane.

If you notice a lump when you are augmenting an area with dermal filler, the first thing to do is assess it to ensure that it is predominantly filler and not just soft tissue oedema or a small haematoma. If it is filler, it should be compressible, elastic and feel similar to the other areas which you have augmented. Oedema will feel like a slightly firm area whereas a haematoma will often present as a dark, palpable bruise which is often tender to touch. Once you have ascertained that there is a filler lump present, the most effective treatment is localised massage. If it is a lump within the lips, then ask your patient to lick their them as saliva makes an effective lubricant to decrease any friction whilst massaging. Should it be within the nasolabial folds then patients can often tolerate massage here without lubrication. Massage the lump between your index finger and thumb to smooth the filler out along the entire tissue plane, using the same technique as in overfilling. The one distinction between managing these two complications in that with acute lumps you needn't "milk" the filler out through puncture sites, you should simply aim to redistribute the filler within the area of augmentation to still create an effective cosmetic outcome. Prompt massage will usually dissipate the filler well within the soft tissues and prevent any hard or long-lasting lumps forming. If you do create a filler lump which you massage at the time of augmentation, then it is advisable for your patient to massage the lump for the next 10 to 14 days. It is beneficial advise to them is to clean their hands thoroughly and, using the technique outlined earlier, to massage their lips twice a day, usually when they have just brushed their teeth (the reason for this being is that it is something done twice daily and therefore they are less likely to forget).

Tiny lumps may not be noticeable at the time of augmentation due to localised oedema and will become visible once the swelling has settled down a few days post-treatment. They are often seen when a patient smiles, laughs or talks in a manner which stretches out overlying tissues. They are most problematic and cosmetically displeasing within the lips, where their off-white colour is demonstrated in stark contrast to the normal pinky-red hues of the lips themselves. If your patient notices these lumps within two weeks of treatment, then you can yet again advise them to massage the area. It is advisable for you to make an urgent appointment to see them to massage the area and teach them to how to do this in person. A face-to-face assessment is also often useful to allow you to exclude these lumps from being a more worrisome condition, such as an infection or abscess. If the lumps do not settle, then you have three realistic choices. The first of which is to wait a few weeks and then re-augment the area in question with the aim of burying the lumps within the new filler. The second is to do nothing and wait for them to dissolve naturally, and the third is to actively remove the lumps which can be via hyaluronidase administration or incision and manual removal of lumps under local anaesthesia.

Some lumps are only noticeable on palpation by the patient but without any associated negative cosmesis. If this is the case and it was just raised in passing by your patient, then it is often advisable to leave them well alone. If it is not causing them any real bother and the area of augmentation looks good then there is no need to perform further interventions which will only serve to increase the risk of infection, anaphylaxis, undesirable cosmesis and so on.

## THE TYNDALL EFFECT

The Tyndall effect is a phenomenon which happens when light is scattered by particles in a colloid solution. As this isn't a physics textbook we shan't dwell on the science behind it too much, just note that in colloid solutions blue light is scattered more greatly than red. This means that clear colloid solutions such as dermal fillers can appear blue. The relevance of this to your cosmetic practice is that dermal fillers are a colloid solution and therefore can develop a bluish hue and discolour the surrounding skin. In the acute phase, the Tyndall effect is often mistaken for a deep bruise; however, the primary discerning feature is that unlike a bruise this will not resolve spontaneously over the next few weeks (Figure 13.4).

There are a few considerations one must make to decrease the chances of the Tyndall effect occurring. The first of which is inserting filler at the correct depth. The more superficial a filler is, the more light that can reach it, and therefore, the greater the potential risk of a bluish discoloration. The second consideration is the volume of filler, as a greater volume of filler will allow more light to scatter and yet again have a greater chance of the Tyndall effect occurring. It is therefore paramount to stress the risk of this when you consent any patients to any filler therapy in which you are likely to insert large boluses.

Regarding patient factors, the Tyndall effect is more likely to occur in areas of thinner tissues, poor-quality skin and in older patients. The anatomical sites where it is most likely to occur are tear troughs, the perioral region and nasolabial folds.

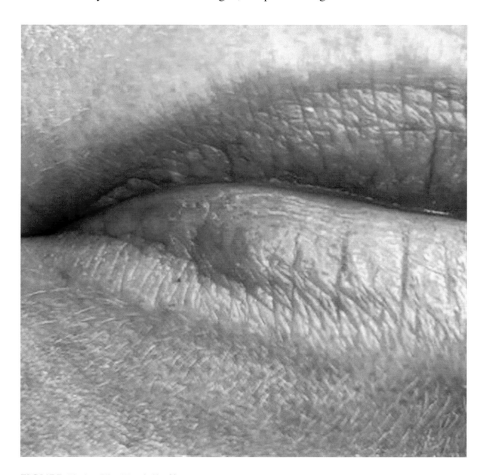

FIGURE 13.4   The Tyndall effect.

Should you have a patient who develops this complication, your first approach should be to massage the area to try and decrease the volume of filler and consequent scatter effect of light. Should that prove to be ineffective the next most sensible approach would be to re-puncture the site with a wide-bore needle and milk the filler out of the skin. Should you fail at both procedures, then you may wish to consider dissolving the filled area with hyaluronidase. Some patients will not find the Tyndall effect bothersome and are happy to cover the area in make-up, so in this cohort, a more passive approach may be best.

## ANAPHYLAXIS

Anaphylaxis is a very real threat to life following administration of any treatment and is even more likely to occur following the use of hyaluronidase as previously discussed. When undertaking any cosmetic procedures in the community, you must have a "grab bag" present on you at all times containing the necessary drugs and airway adjuncts to save a patient's life should this occur. Due to the severity of an anaphylactic reaction, it is always worth ensuring that you have sufficient training in advanced life support and that you do not let your certification expire, no matter how experienced you are.

In order to successfully be able to manage a case of anaphylaxis, you must first understand the mechanism of hypersensitivity reactions and their physiological effects on the body. Philip Gell and Robin Coombs first proposed the classification system of hypersensitivity reactions in 1963, a system which is still used today (Table 13.7).

## TABLE 13.7
### The Gell and Coombs Hypersensitivity Classification System

| Type | Examples | Mediators | Effects |
|---|---|---|---|
| I (Allergy) | Atopy Allergy Anaphylaxis | Immunoglobulin E (IgE) | Type I reactions occur in seconds to minutes from the allergen triggering a hypersensitivity response. Antigens cross-link IgE on mast cells and basophils, initiating a release of molecules such as histamine. |
| II (Cytotoxic) | Thrombocytopaenia Goodpasture's syndrome Autoimmune haemolytic anaemia | IgM/IgG Complement cascade Membrane Attack Complex (MAC) | Antibodies bind to antigens on native cells which the body perceives as foreign. This causes resultant cellular destruction via the MAC. |
| III (Immune Complex) | Rheumatoid arthritis Systemic lupus erythematosus Hypersensitivity pneumonitis | IgG Complement cascade Neutrophils | IgG binds to the circulating antigen and forms an immune complex. This is then deposited in tiny capillaries causing a localised immune reaction at these sites. |
| IV (Cell-Mediated) | Contact dermatitis Coeliac disease Chronic transplant rejection | T cells | Th1 cells become activated by an antigen. With future exposure, Th1 cells activate macrophages and trigger an aberrant inflammatory response. |

Please note, there is also a fifth type of hypersensitivity reaction, which is similar in nature to Type V. The primary distinction between Type II and Type V hypersensitivity reactions is that in Type V reactions antibodies bind to cell surface receptors and inhibit cell signalling. Examples of type V hypersensitivity reactions include Grave's disease and Myasthenia Gravis.

Type I hypersensitivity reactions are our primary cause for concern in the acute phase with dermal filler augmentation, and it is essential to understand the chain of events which, if untreated, can result in a fatal anaphylactic reaction.

### PATHOPHYSIOLOGY OF ANAPHYLAXIS

Anaphylaxis is a Type I hypersensitivity reaction and is in essence a severe allergic reaction causing systemic compromise which requires the presence of immunoglobulin E (IgE) antibodies being exposed to a particular allergen. Inevitably, every single one of us will at some point or another have IgE antibodies exposed to allergens; however, only about one in 1,000 people will ever experience a true anaphylactic reaction, suggesting there are likely a set of risk factors which make an individual more likely to develop anaphylaxis. It has been noted that a history of atopy may make an individual more likely to experience such a reaction, with asthma in particular being associated with increased mortality. It is unclear, however, if there is true causation between asthma and the severity of anaphylaxis, and it may just be that they are more likely to suffer life-threatening bronchospasm.

The first step of an anaphylactic reaction is the binding of IgE to the offending antigen. The antigen-bound IgE then activates FcεRI receptors on mast cells, basophils and eosinophils initiating a process known as *degranulation*. Mast cells are strategically positioned within the upper and lower respiratory tract, beneath the skin and within the gastrointestinal tract; giving them the best opportunity to intercept antigens which we touch, inhale or ingest.

*Granules* are secretory vesicles which are found within the cytoplasm of cells. They act as a storage unit for substances to be used at a later date, and the granule allows them to be kept in an inert manner before being released into the extracellular environment when required.

*Degranulation* is, in essence, the release of said granular contents from within a cell to its surrounding environment. Regarding anaphylaxis, the mechanism of release is through a *tyrosine-kinase phosphorylation cascade* after a pro-inflammatory cell (such as a mast cell) has been activated by an IgE-antigen complex. The relevance of a phosphorylation cascade is that through enzymatic phosphorylation a small signal can be rapidly and significantly amplified via a short series of chemical reactions. This phosphorylation cascade results in an influx in intracellular calcium, which in itself is the trigger for degranulation to occur. When mast cells degranulate, they release pro-inflammatory mediators such as histamine, prostaglandin and cytokines such as TNF-α. See Figure 13.5.

The combined effect of the release of pro-inflammatory cytokines is peripheral vasodilation, smooth muscle contraction, pulmonary vasoconstriction and increased capillary permeability. In anaphylaxis, the overall effect of this is a tight throat, swollen mucous membranes and decreased blood supply to vital organs. In short,

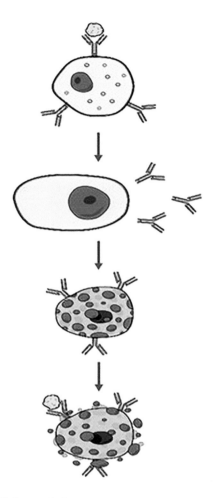

**FIGURE 13.5**    Mast cell degranulation.

it is the release of these tiny chemical mediators which is responsible for the life-threatening consequences of anaphylactic shock.

### SIGNS AND SYMPTOMS OF ANAPHYLAXIS

Anaphylaxis can present within seconds to minutes of exposure to an allergen. Signs and symptoms of an anaphylactic reaction include the following:

- Facial flushing
- Sweating
- Facial swelling
- Swelling of the lips and tongue

- Urticaria
- Wheeze
- Hypotension
- Tachycardia
- Tachypnoea
- Warm and clammy extremities

Anaphylaxis may kill patients via a combination of two cascading events. The first of which is through airway occlusion secondary to both oedema of the airways and bronchospasm. The second is that histamine release causes systemic vasodilation and consequent hypotension, which can result in anaphylactic shock. A combination of these two pathways has a significant chance of resulting in a fatal outcome.

## MANAGEMENT OF ANAPHYLAXIS

Prompt recognition and treatment of anaphylaxis saves lives. You need to commit the signs, symptoms and management of anaphylaxis to memory so you can effectively treat it and prevent a tragic outcome.

If a patient complains of itching, chest tightness, tongue swelling, wheezing, or difficulty breathing whilst you are undertaking a procedure, then you should stop immediately to prevent the administration of an increased volume of the allergen in question. Take a moment to assess your patient for the aforementioned symptoms, and if you should suspect an anaphylactic reaction, then waste no time in calling for help. Try to get the attention of anybody nearby and instruct them to call an ambulance and inform the emergency services that you have a patient who is having an anaphylactic reaction.

Always ensure you have an anaphylaxis pack with you whenever performing any cosmetic treatments. Ensure you regularly audit your equipment and drugs to ensure that they are fully functional and within date. Should you need to use any equipment from the pack, re-order it and do not provide any treatments until you have your pack reassembled and properly organised (Figure 13.6). Failure to have a properly stocked and maintained anaphylaxis pack can result in fatal consequences.

### ANAPHYLAXIS PACK CONTENTS

- ✓ Oxygen cylinder
- ✓ Non-rebreathe mask
- ✓ Adrenaline 0.5 ml 1:1000 solution (Always have at least two)
- ✓ Green cannula and saline flush
- ✓ 200 mg hydrocortisone and 10 mg chlorphenamine IV
- ✓ 1 L normal saline

FIGURE 13.6   Sample contents of a standard anaphylaxis pack.

Even if your patient makes a full initial recovery as a result of your treatment, they must still go to hospital. This is because there is a risk of "rebound anaphylaxis" once the adrenaline has been metabolised. As in the case of infections, when your patient is taken to hospital, write a brief letter for their clinicians so they know exactly what cosmetic treatments you have performed and the drugs and doses you have used to treat their anaphylactic reaction. You should also contact your cosmetic supplier to inform them of the batch number of the product used so they can undertake their own investigation. Finally, don't forget to replenish your "grab bag" of oxygen, salbutamol, adrenaline, hydrocortisone and chlorphenamine.

## LATE COMPLICATIONS: DELAYED-ONSET NODULES

Delayed-onset nodules are essentially a new nodularity or mass at or adjacent to the site of injection. These nodules are most likely to present a few months after treatment and if untreated can be psychologically distressing for your patients. The probability of developing a delayed onset nodule can be broken down into patient, practitioner and product factors. These may have an aggregative effect should there be an inappropriate patient injected in a technically poor manner with an unsuitable filler for the treated anatomical location.

Delayed onset nodules are hypothesised to be a Type IV autoimmune reactions and therefore are more likely to occur in patients with a history of hypersensitivity reactions such as asthma and atopic eczema. Care should also be taken with any patient with an autoimmune condition such as systemic lupus erythematosus or rheumatoid arthritis due to this theoretical risk. Delayed-onset nodules have also been reported to have a higher incidence in highly mobile areas such as the lips or perioral region.

Unsurprisingly, the rate of delayed onset nodules (and, indeed, any complication) is decreased when the procedure is performed by an experienced practitioner with an in-depth knowledge of the relevant anatomy and correct injection technique. Filler injected too superficially greatly increases the risk of filler nodule formation, as does using an inappropriately thick filler in the superficial dermis or epidermis. The area treated also raises certain risks of delayed onset nodule formation, with more mobile areas and those with less subcutaneous tissue conferring a greater risk. The composition of dermal filler may also present as an independent risk factor, as particulate gels appear to create a greater local inflammatory response and are subsequently more likely to result in delayed onset nodule formation. One final consideration to make is regarding bolus injection of filler. Fibrous capsules may form around large boluses of dermal filler on the surface which is exposed to the surrounding soft tissues. These capsules may then scar and contract forming a potentially painful nodule in this location.

The lips are one of the most likely places to develop nodule formation, which may be due to the thin dermal layer, high levels of bacterial flora and the strong, hypermobile underlying muscle. Another area of caution is filling in the periorbital region due to complex vascular, lymphatic and nervous anatomy with bony prominences, relative paucity of overlying fat and thin skin. This region is therefore only advisable for treatment by experienced practitioners with a good grasp of the relevant anatomy.

Delayed-onset nodules can be broken down into inflammatory and non-inflammatory nodules, which are discussed in further detail next.

### Non-inflammatory nodules

This may well be somewhat of a misnomer as noninflammatory nodules have been hypothesised to be a low-grade, chronic inflammatory response to dermal filler augmentation. The greatest risk factor for non-inflammatory nodule formation is filler deposition in an incorrect anatomical plane or the use of an inappropriate filler for the location treated. Non-inflammatory nodules are stereotypically characterised by a firm, well-circumscribed smooth nodule which is neither tender nor warm on palpation. If these nodules are superficial, they may also be visible are and will be pale in comparison to the surrounding skin.

The management of non-inflammatory nodules is often determined by their size. Small nodules can often be treated by injection at the site of treatment with saline or lidocaine of the same volume of filler used. This technique will displace the nodule and hopefully disperse it within the local soft tissues. Another approach is to use a 21G needle to excise and aspirate the nodule itself. Larger nodules, however, may require dissolving with hyaluronidase should they prove bothersome to your patient. If your attempts prove fruitless in rectifying the problem, then you may wish to rethink your diagnosis as your patient may have an inflammatory nodule instead.

### Inflammatory nodules

One of the key discriminating factors for inflammatory compared to non-inflammatory nodules is their frequent presentation with pain and erythema. The current consensus as to the formation of inflammatory nodules is that the treated area becomes contaminated with a low-grade, chronic infection. The introduction of these infections may be either due to contaminated filler or direct inoculation with skin commensals at the time of treatment. Inflammatory nodules may prove difficult to treat as there is evidence to suggest that causative bacteria may secrete a polymeric jacket to protect themselves from the immune system and antibiotic agents. The bacteria may then lay dormant for an indeterminate period until the local environment proves favourable for replication, like an animal hibernating over winter. Once the bacteria awaken they may then develop into granulomatous inflammation, abscesses, or inflammatory nodules.

Please be aware that the management of noninflammatory nodules should only be undertaken by an experienced practitioner with advanced training in the management of dermal filler complications. There is no shame in referring your patient to a consultant dermatologist or plastic surgeon should you believe that you have reached the level of your expertise. Prompt referral confers the best possible outcome for your patient both cosmetically and holistically.

Initial management of an inflammatory nodule is with antibiotics. Sensible choices would be clarithromycin 500 mg BD and/or tetracycline 100 mg BD for four weeks. Should your patient have an allergy to these agents then a potential third-line antibiotic may be ciprofloxacin 500 mg BD for two weeks; however, ciprofloxacin confers an increased risk of pseudomembranous colitis, Achilles tendon rupture, and cardiac arrythmias. It may be prudent to initially start your patient on dual-antibiotic therapy for four weeks and then re-review them to ensure they are clinically improving.

Should your patient not improve after four weeks of antibiotic therapy, then consider dissolving the nodule with hyaluronidase. You may wish to continue the course of antibiotics at your discretion whilst undertaking hyaluronidase treatment. Should there be a benefit with hyaluronidase then you may wish to repeat dissolution at four-weekly intervals until they have fully resolved. Should you fail to garner a successful outcome after hyaluronidase administration then you should explore other management options.

Management of inflammatory nodules refractory to treatment involves intralesional steroid injection and/or initiating allopurinol and continuation of antibiotics dependent on the clinical judgement of the assessing practitioner. It is worth noting that common side effects of steroid treatment are localised tissue atrophy, discoloration and *worsening* of the underlying infection or abscess. Other radical treatments may include localised heat therapy with lasers or via radiofrequency ablation. Should all else fail, surgical excision may be necessitated by an experienced doctor or surgeon in a formal operating theatre.

## PERSISTENT SWELLING

As previously discussed, swelling after dermal filler augmentation usually peaks the morning after treatment and lasts for two days to two weeks. In some cases, however, patients may develop post-procedural swelling later than the first post-treatment day which persists for much longer than expected. The swelling may encompass the entire region treated or just a portion of it. Despite being a benign phenomenon, it can be quite distressing to both the practitioner and patient as the primary treatment is to simply do nothing at all.

As with all complications, it is strongly advisable to review any patient reporting persisting swelling as a matter of urgency to assess for any potential underlying infection or reaction to the filler itself. Persistent swelling is almost always painless; however, it may be slightly tender to touch but nowhere near as painful as an abscess or cellulitis. Once you are happy that the patient does not have a serious underlying pathology, you can explain to them that this swelling will likely settle over the coming weeks (in the author's experience, this process may take up to a month to fully resolve). This watch-and-wait strategy requires a significant amount of trust in both a patient–practitioner manner as well as the practitioner trusting their clinical acumen sufficiently! Ask your patient to take photographs on a weekly basis and to send them to you so you can monitor the swelling decreasing in size. Should it not settle after two months, then it is most likely that you have overfilled the area as opposed to it simply being post-procedural swelling. In these instances, you should be honest with your patient that this is the most likely diagnosis and address asymmetry as previously discussed in the section detailing the management of overfilling earlier in this chapter.

Figure 13.7 shows is a series of photographs detailing the dramatic effects of delayed and persistent post-procedural swelling. The photographs were taken

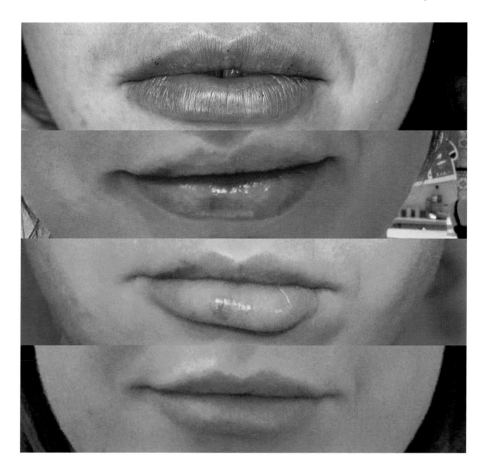

**FIGURE 13.7**    Persistent swelling after lip augmentation.

immediately after the treatment, day two post-treatment, one week post-treatment and at one month. The swelling fully dissipated by six weeks with an even contour to the lip and a satisfactory cosmetic outcome.

## LATE COMPLICATIONS: FOREIGN BODY GRANULOMAS

Foreign body granulomas often present as sterile erythematous nodules, plaques or papules which may or may not be ulcerated. They are a relatively common inflammatory complication to dermal filler injection and are part of the immune response of the body to isolate a foreign body which cannot be immediately rectified by an enzymatic or phagocytotic response. Inflammatory mediators stimulate encapsulation of the foreign body by both monocytes and macrophages. Upon failing to phagocytose the material, macrophages secrete proinflammatory cytokines to attract greater numbers of macrophages and monocytes to wall off the alien substance.

Macrophages may also differentiate into epithelioid histiocytes or foreign body giant cells, which are pathognomic to granulomata and exhibit a granulomatous reaction histologically.

Granuloma formation may occur in as many as one in one hundred dermal filler treatments and may have an extended dormant period of months to years after treatment. Accurate documentation at the time of the injection procedure and product at the time of treatment will prove invaluable in their diagnosis and management should they develop in the future. The development of a granuloma is more likely in patients who have a larger volume of filler, fillers containing microparticles, previous infection at the site of infection and direct trauma to the region of augmentation. They are also theorised to be more prominent in patients with high-circulating IgE and atopic conditions such as asthma and eczema.

As in the treatment of inflammatory delayed onset nodules, the management of a foreign body granuloma should only be managed by an experienced practitioner who is appropriately trained in the conservative and surgical management of these nodules. Initial therapy is recommended as intralesional steroid injection. Concomitant hyaluronidase therapy may also be useful in dissolving the granulomatous component. Should conservative management fail, the next step is surgical excision of the foreign body and its surrounding granulomatous capsule. If the patient still wants further treatment then this should only be performed in an operating theatre by an experienced doctor or surgeon due to the risk of post-operative infection and scar formation.

# Bibliography

Akinbiyi T., et al., "Better Results in Facial Rejuvenation with Fillers" *International Open Access Journal of the American Society of Plastic Surgeons* 2020 Oct; 8(10): 2763.

Berman A., Chutka D., "Assessing Effective Physician-Patient Communication Skills: 'Are You Listening to Me, Doc?'" *Korean Journal of Medical Education* 2016 Jun; 28(2): 243–249.

Bjorksten J., "The Crosslinking Theory of Aging" *Journal of the American Geriatrics Society* 1968 Apr; 16(4): 408–427.

Bjorksten J., Tenhu H., "The Crosslinking Theory of Aging: Added Evidence" *Experimental Geronotology* 1990; 25(2): 91–95.

Boss G., Seegmiller J., "Age-Related Physiological Changes and Their Clinical Significance" *Western Journal of Medicine* 1981 Dec; 135(6): 434–440.

Byrd A., Belkaid Y., Segre J., "The Human Skin Microbiome" *Nature Reviews Microbiology* 2018 Jan; 16: 143–155.

Canedo-Dorantes L., Canedo-Ayala M., "Skin Acute Wound Healing: A Comprehensive Review" *International Journal of Inflammation* 2019 Jun; 10: 1155.

Chatterjee N., Walker G., "Mechanisms of DNA Repair and Mutagenesis" *Environmental and Molecular Mutagenesis* 2017 May; 58(5): 235–263.

Choon P.D., Geun Y.S., "Aging" *Korean Journal of Audiology* 2013 Sep; 17(2): 39–44.

Farage M., et al., "Intrinsic and Extrinsic Factors in Skin Ageing: A Review" *International Journal of Cosmetic Sciences* 2008 Mar; 30(2): 87–95.

Francheschi C., et al., "The Continuum of Aging and Age-Related Diseases: Common Mechanisms But Different Rates" *Frontiers in Medicine* 2018 Mar; 5(61).

Funt D., Pavacic T., "Dermal Fillers in Aesthetics: An Overview of Adverse Events and Treatment Approaches" *Clinical, Cosmetic and Investigational Dermatology* 2013 Dec; 6: 295–316.

Ganceviciene R., "Skin Anti-Aging Strategies" *Dermato Endocrinology* 2012 Jul; 4(3): 308–319.

Ibanez-Berganza M., et al., "Subjectivity and Complexity of Facial Attractiveness" *Nature Scientific Reports* 2019 Jun; 8364.

Jin K., "Modern Biological Theories of Aging" *Aging and Disease* 2010 Oct; 1(2): 72–74.

Kassir M., et al., "Complications of Botulinum Toxin and Fillers: A Narrative Review" *Journal of Cosmetic Dermatology* 19(3): 570–573.

Kee J., et al., "Communication Skills in Patient-Doctor Interactions: Learning from Patient Complaints" *Heath Professions Education* 2018 Jun; 4(2): 97–106.

Kennedy S., Loeb L., Herr A., "Somatic Mutations in Aging, Cancer and Neurodegeneration" *Mechanisms of Aging and Development* 2012 Apr; 133(4): 118–126.

Kraft-Todd G., et al., "Empathetic Nonverbal Behaviour Increases Ratings of Both Warmth and Competence in a Medical Context" *PLoS One* 2017 May; 12(5): 1–16.

Langan S., et al., "Atopic Dermatitis" *The Lancet* 2020 Apr; 396(10247): 345–360.

Langlois J., Roggman L., "Attractive Faces Are Only Average" *Psychological Science* 1990 Mar; 1(2): 115–121.

Little A., et al., "Facial Attractiveness: Evolutionary Based Research" *Philosophical Transactions of the Royal Society* B 2011 Jun; 366(1571): 1638–1659.

MacNee W., Rabinovich R., Choudhury G., "Ageing and the Border between Health and Disease" *European Respiratory Journal* 2014; 44: 1332–1352.

McMasters K., "Evaluation of Malignant and Premalignant Skin Lesions" in Bland K.I., et al., eds., *General Surgery* (2nd edn) Springer Reference 2009 1569–1578.

Nestor M., Arnold D., Fischer D., "The Mechanisms of Action and Use of Botulinum Neurotoxin Type A in Aesthetics: Key Clinical Postulates II" *Journal of Cosmetic Dermatology* 2020 19(11): 2785–2804.

Pirazzini M., et al., "Botulinum Neurotoxins: Biology, Pharmacology, and Toxicology" *Pharmacology Reviews* 2017 Apr; 69(2): 200–235.

Prinzinger R., "Programmed Ageing: The Theory of Maximal Metabolic Scope" *EMBO Reports* 2005 Jul; 6: 14–19.

Raje N., Dinakar C., "Overview of Immunodeficiency Disorders" *Immunology and Allergy Clinics of North America* 2015 Nov; 35(4): 599–623.

Rashid S., Ngee Shim T., "Contact Dermatitis" *British Medical Journal* 2016 Jun; 353.

Rendon A., Schakel K., "Psoriasis Pathogenesis and Treatment" *International Journal of Molecular Sciences* 2019 Mar; 20(6): 1475.

Rohrich R., Bartlett E., Dayan E., "Practical Approach and Safety of Hyaluronic Acid Fillers" *Plastic and Reconstructive Surgery: Global Open* 2019 Jun; 7(6): 2172.

Russell-Goldnam E., Murphy G., "The Pathobiology of Skin Ageing: New Insights into an Old Dilemma" *American Journal of Pathology* 2020 Apr; 190(7): 1356–1369.

Silverman J., Kinnersley P., "Doctors' Non-Verbal Behaviour in Consultations: Look at the Patient before You Look at the Computer" *British Journal of General Practice* 2010 Feb; 60(571): 76–78.

van Deursen J., "The Role of Senescent Cells in Ageing" *Nature* 2014 May; 509(7501): 439–446.

van Heemst D., "Insulin, IGF-1 and Longevity" *Aging and Disease* 2010 Oct; 1(2): 147–157.

Wan D., et al., "The Clinical Importance of the Fat Compartments in Midfacial Aging" *PRS Global Open* 2014 Jan; 1(9): 92.

Williams C., et al., "Acne Vulgaris" *The Lancet* 2012 Feb; 361–172.

Wollina U., Goldman A., Tchernev G., "Fillers and Facial Fat Pads" *Open Access Macedonian Journal of Medical Sciences* 2017 Jul; 5(4): 403–408.

# Index

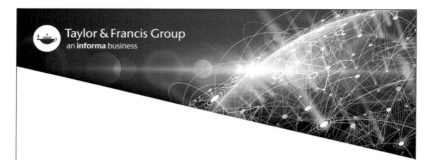